An Illustrated Pocketbook of Multiple Sclerosis

Charles M. Poser, MD, FRCP, DMS
Department of Neurology,
Harvard Medical School and Beth Israel
Deaconess Medical Center, Boston, MA, USA

The Parthenon Publishing Group
International Publishers in Medicine, Science & Technology

A CRC PRESS COMPANY

BOCA RATON   LONDON   NEW YORK   WASHINGTON, D.C.

Published in the USA by
The Parthenon Publishing Group
345 Park Avenue South, 10th Floor
New York, NY 10010, USA

Published in the UK and Europe by
The Parthenon Publishing Group Limited
23–25 Blades Court
Deodar Road
London SW15 2NU, UK

Library of Congress Cataloging-in-Publication Data
Data available on application

British Library Cataloguing in Publication Data
Poser, Charles M.
 An illustrated pocketbook of multiple sclerosis
 1. Multiple sclerosis - Diagnosis 2. Multiple sclerosis
 Treatment
 I. Title
 618.9'29

ISBN 1-84214-141-4

Copyright © 2003 The Parthenon Publishing Group

Contents

Introduction 7

Epidemiology and genetics 9

Etiology 12

Pathogenesis 13

Pathology 25

Physiology 39

Clinical aspects 40
Clinical course 41

Diagnosis 44
Diagnostic criteria 44
The new MS diagnostic criteria of McDonald 45
Optic fundus and visual fields 45
Confirmatory laboratory procedures 47
Examination of cerebrospinal fluid 47
Evoked potential studies 53
Neuroimaging 55
Magnetic resonance imaging 59
Imaging differential diagnoses 68
Single photon emission computed tomography 86
Positron emission tomography 87

Treatment 89

Conclusion 90

Bibliography 91

Index 97

Introduction

Multiple sclerosis (MS) has fascinated physicians ever since it was first described. Its extraordinary clinical variability and its unpredictability, when added to the complexities of the immune system alterations believed to play an important role in its development, may explain why it has attracted such great interest. Its importance is underlined by the fact that it affects two million people world-wide. The disease has been known for over 160 years but, despite enormous expenditures of time and money on research, many aspects of its pathogenesis are still unknown.

There is, as yet, no clear understanding of the etiology and risk factors, and of the meaning of much epidemiological data. Most importantly, fully effective modes of prevention and treatment remain elusive. Because it affects men and women in their most productive time of life, and may cause the end of a promising career or a happy marriage, it is often viewed as a devastating illness that can rarely be helped with treatment. Most acute bouts can be rapidly and effectively terminated and there are many symptomatic measures available that can significantly improve the comfort and quality of life of patients with MS. Long-term treatment has now become available, but, while these drugs reduce the number of relapses, it is not yet clear if they have a significant effect on the progress of the disease. Fortunately, only a minority of patients are rendered severely disabled by the disease. There is still much to be learned about MS, but progress has been made, particularly in regard to the reliability of available diagnostic methods, as well as our understanding of its pathology.

Multiple sclerosis is an acute inflammatory disease that causes focal demyelination of the brain and spinal cord; it also causes axonal loss. There is evidence for limited remyelination of indeterminate significance. The disease is characterized by dissemination in space and time. The lesions involve separate parts of the central nervous system

7

and thus signs and symptoms cannot be ascribed to a single lesion. In addition, its clinical course is most often characterized by exacerbations and remissions. The usual age of onset is in the third or fourth decade. In that age group, MS is second only to epilepsy as the most common disease of the central nervous system (CNS). With rare exceptions, MS does not involve the peripheral nervous system.

Epidemiology and genetics

Multiple sclerosis is not evenly distributed throughout the world. For many years, it had been suggested that the prevalence of MS, in Europe in particular, was directly related to latitude: the further from the equator, the more common the disease. However, wide variations in prevalence between geographical areas of similar latitude prove this idea to be incorrect, except for the yet unexplained observations that Tasmania has a prevalence of MS twice that of southern Australia, despite the fact that the populations in these two areas have essentially identical ethnic origins.

The north–south gradient that has been repeatedly demonstrated in the United States is derived from the fact that the proportion of multiple sclerosis patients in the population of people of Scandinavian descent, who seem to have a special susceptibility, is considerably higher in the northern tier of states than in the southern. A similar gradient, but at a somewhat lower level of prevalence, is apparent in black American MS patients (Figure 1). This may also be explained by the existence of a gradient, going from the south to the north, that shows an increasing admixture of Caucasian genetic material in black Americans, as measured by blood groups.

Three independent epidemiological studies of MS in immigrants to South Africa, Hawaii and the West Coast of the United States have all indicated that the disease is acquired some time before puberty. Therefore, putative dates of acquisition rather than dates of clinical onset of the disease are more important. This is well illustrated by the reports of epidemics of MS. Epidemics of MS are said to have occurred in Iceland and in the Faroe Islands as a result of a cryptic infection brought by British troops during World War II, but recalculation of the data on the basis of age of acquisition revealed that the peak incidence occurred before the arrival of these troops. This has not prevented the

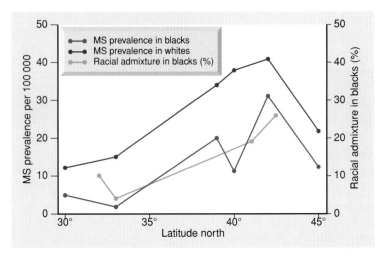

Figure 1 Prevalence of multiple sclerosis in blacks compared with whites in the USA. Note that the percentage of racial admixture in blacks, based on blood group studies, parallels the rate of prevalence in blacks. Modified from Poser, 1992; reproduced with the permission of Elsevier Science BV

repeated references to these alleged epidemics in textbooks and articles.

Racial or ethnic origin plays an important, but not exclusive, role in determining susceptibility to the disease. No convincingly documented cases of MS have ever been reported in North and South American Indians, Eskimos, Lapps, Australian aborigines, Maoris, Polynesians, Melanesians, and Micronesians. The disease occurs much less frequently in Orientals and extremely rarely in black Africans. Because of these indications, numerous studies of genetic markers have been carried out but, to date, few secure candidates or regions have been identified. Many studies of the class II major histocompatibility complex (MHC) alleles of the human leukocyte antigen (HLA) system and their genotypes have been carried out. Some of these have suggested an association between the MHC alleles DR15 and DQ6 (DRB1*1501 and DBQ2 *0602) and the gene for tissue necrosis factor encoded within the same linkage group. A specifically different association (with DR4 and its DRB1*0405-DQA1*0301-DQB1*0302 genotype) is seen in Mediterranean populations, primarily Sardinians.

There is a familial occurrence rate of about 15%. The age-adjusted risk is higher in siblings (3%), parents (2%), and children (2%) than for second- and third-degree relatives. There is only a 35% concordance in monozygotic twins, but it is the same as in siblings for dizygotic pairs. Children of conjugal pairs with MS have a much higher rate (20%), but adopted offspring or other non-biological relatives have no increased risk. There is strong evidence to suggest that MS is a polygenic disease.

In addition to the crucial genetic factor, there is also an important environmental influence. This has been shown by a number of reliable investigations such as the one that showed that Frenchmen living in Africa have a considerably lower prevalence rate compared with Frenchmen living in France. The children of West Indian and Asian immigrants to the United Kingdom are said to have the same levels of incidence and prevalence as native-born Englishmen, and the Israel-born children of both Ashkenazi and Sephardic Jews appear to have the same prevalence rates, although the European-born parents of the former have a much higher prevalence rate than the Asian and African-born parents of the latter. The situation in Hawaii illustrates what appears to be the interplay between genetic and environmental influences. For subjects of Japanese extraction living in either Hawaii or the mainland United States, the environment appears to increase the risk of acquiring MS compared with that of those living in Japan. For Caucasians, however, being raised in or moving to Hawaii appears to offer some protection against MS. This strongly supports the idea that environmental factors vary from place to place and affect susceptible populations in different ways. A large number of studies on an enormous variety of possible agents and factors that could conceivably influence the acquisition or development of the disease have been carried out in many countries, with an almost total lack of results. Most of the agents and factors are really meaningless since they are completely lacking in biological plausibility. In summary, epidemiological studies have demonstrated the primary importance of genetic factors modified by as yet unrecognized environmental influences.

Etiology

Multiple sclerosis has been described as 'a disease of unknown etiology', implying the existence of a single causal organism. A number of infectious agents have been reported as potential etiological agents. They include the corona, measles, Epstein–Barr, herpes simplex type 6, and canine distemper viruses, the human T-cell lymphotrophic virus (HTLV)-I, an 'MS-associated agent' and, most recently, *Chlamydia*. None of these has been confirmed, but the idea lingers on, despite exhaustive searches by competent investigators using sophisticated techniques. From all of the information that is currently available on the disease, it is much more likely that MS is the result, in a genetically susceptible subject, of the activation of the immune system by different viral agents, thereby initiating a pathogenetic cascade that eventually leads to the destruction of the myelin sheath and the axon. Many steps in this process remain unknown.

Pathogenesis

The precise pathogenetic mechanism of MS remains controversial, but many investigators believe that alterations of the immune system are responsible. It is likely that some of these changes are, in fact, the result of the disease process rather than its cause, or that they co-exist. The vast majority of investigators believe that the pathogenetic process can be initiated only by an immunological event altering the impermeability of the blood–brain barrier (Figures 2 and 3). There is evidence to suggest that other, non-specific events and factors, such as electrical injury, lipid solvents and trauma, can do the same. This is *not* to say that the latter ever *cause* MS.

Several pathogenetic schemes have been offered, including that proposed by the author (Figure 4). The surprisingly low concordance rate of a disease, with a strong genetic component in monozygotic twins, suggests that what is genetically determined is a premorbid state that the author has called the 'MS trait' (MST), analogous to that in sickle cell disease and glucose-6-phosphate dehydrogenase deficiency. The trait is a systemic non-pathological condition, 'a disease waiting to happen'. At present, not all of the components of the MST have been defined nor can it be detected in the parents, siblings or children of MS patients.

Constituents of the MST include a vigorous antibody response to a great variety of viral antigens, and inflammatory infiltration of the capillaries of the brain parenchyma. This does not lead to changes in the myelin sheaths, but results in minor alterations of the blood–brain barrier that cannot be demonstrated by gadolinium-enhanced magnetic resonance imaging (MRI), but may allow B-lymphocytes to penetrate into the CNS, where they produce oligoclonal bands. These changes have been demonstrated in the normal white matter of MS patients by histoimmunological methods, and, more recently, by special MRI techniques. The enhanced antibody response to many

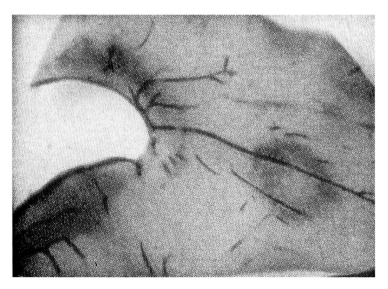

Figure 2 Post-mortem perfusion study of a brain from a patient with multiple sclerosis. The plaques are traversed by venules (stained red). The periphery is stained blue, demonstrating increased permeability of the blood–brain barrier. Supravital trypan blue stain. Courtesy of Professor Töre Broman, University of Göteborg, Sweden

viruses and the presence of oligoclonal bands in the cerebrospinal fluid (CSF) have been found in healthy siblings, including the non-affected monozygotic twins of MS patients.

The MST is the result of a viral antigenic challenge in a genetically susceptible person from either an infection or a vaccine. Such a challenge is non-specific: it may be in the form of measles in one subject, an adenovirus in another, and a vaccination against hepatitis B in a third. This initial challenge to the immune system appears to lead primarily to a response of the B-lymphocytes that produce antibodies and oligoclonal bands in the cerebrospinal fluid. The mechanism of the resulting vasculopathy is unknown, but it most probably increases the vulnerability of the blood–brain barrier. At the stage of the MST, the parenchyma of the CNS remains intact. The MS disease may never develop in a subject with the MST.

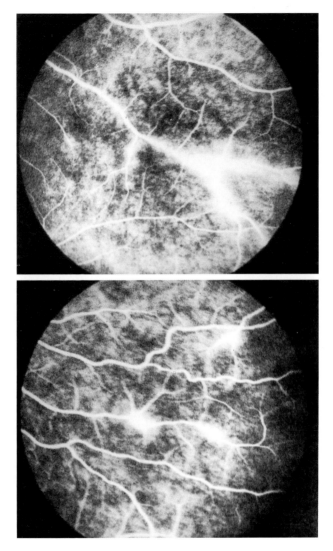

Figure 3 Retinal fluorescein angiography in optic neuritis. Note leakage from vessels, indicating alteration of permeability of the vessel walls in the retina, a myelin-free structure. From Lightman *et al.*, 1987; reproduced with permission of Oxford University Press

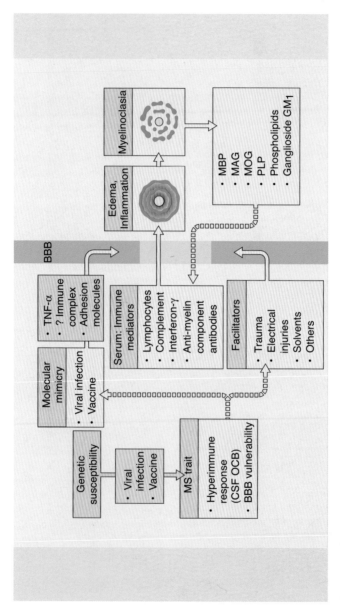

Figure 4 Pathogenesis of multiple sclerosis. BBB, blood–brain barrier; TNF-α, tumor necrosis factor-α; OCB, oligoclonal bands; MBP, myelin basic protein; MAG, myelin-associated glycoprotein; MOG, myelin-oligodendroglia glycoprotein; PLP, proteolipid protein. Modified from Poser, 1994b; reproduced with the permission of John Wiley & Sons

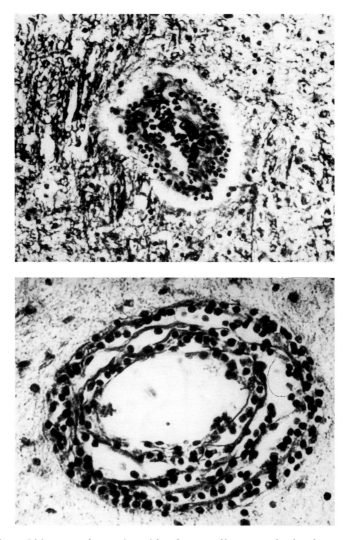

Figure 5 Microscopy showing (upper) lymphocytic infiltration confined to the venous wall in normal white matter in active multiple sclerosis (MS), and (lower) lymphocytic infiltration and edematous onion-skin changes in the venous wall in normal white matter approximately 1.5 cm from an active MS plaque. From Adams *et al.*, 1985; reproduced with permission of Elsevier Science BV

17

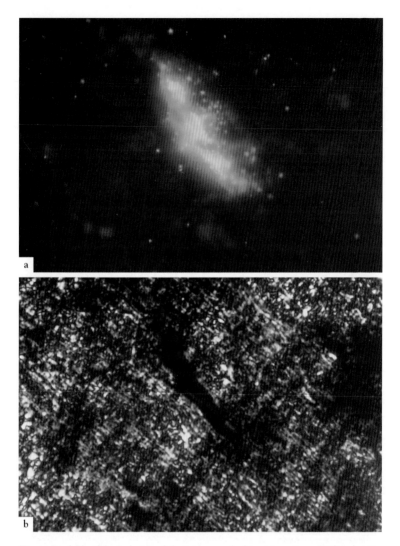

Figure 6a–d Blood–brain barrier defects in normal white matter in multiple sclerosis: (a) Section prepared with rabbit antihuman fibrinogen–tetramethyl rhodamine iso-thiocyanate (TRITC) fluorescein shows fibrinogen leaking from capillary; (b) same section viewed under polarized light shows normal myelin birefringence except in the vessel walls (*continued*)

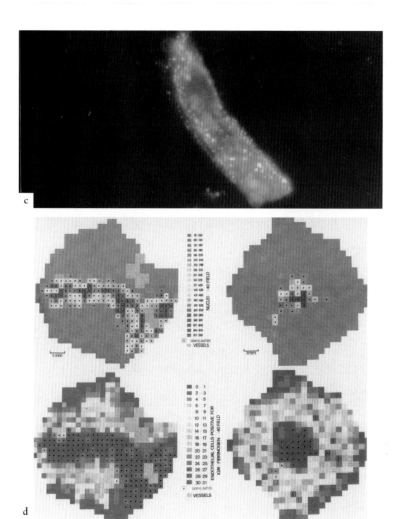

Figure 6 *Continued* (c) capillary endothelial cells containing vesicles positive for IgM fluorescein isothiocyanate (FITC); (d) distribution of BBB abnormalities associated with two acute plaques. The plaques are defined by their hypercellularity (nuclear counts, upper) and myelin lysis (dotted areas). Both plaques (lower) are surrounded by zones of perivascular fibrinogen leakage (see a) and endothelial cell endocytosis of IgM (see c). From Gay and Esiri, 1991, reproduced with the permission of Oxford University Press. For technical details, see Gay *et al.*, 1997

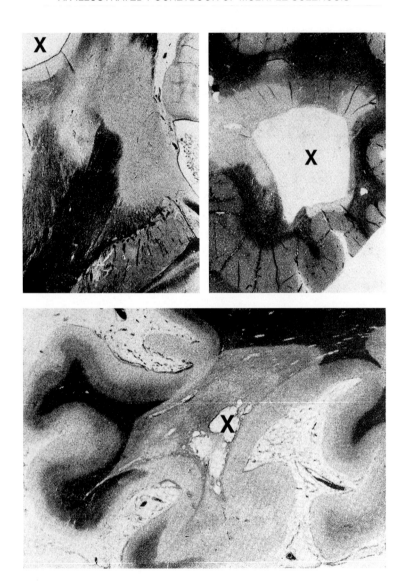

Figure 7 New multiple sclerosis plaques adjacent to brain needle tract (marked by the X), the result of gross breach of the blood–brain barrier. Courtesy of Dr Richard Gonsette, Brussels, Belgium

It is generally accepted that a major alteration of the blood–brain barrier is the first step that leads to the development of the MS lesion. A key role has been suggested for tumor necrosis factor, immune complexes and adhesion molecules. The stimulus for this immunological response is probably a second antigenic challenge from either an infection or a vaccination, but not necessarily by the same agent that led to the MST. Activation of the immune system is through molecular mimicry. This is a phenomenon in which some component peptides of the active antigenic molecule are immunologically indistinguishable from a myelin antigen, and hence an appropriate response to infection generates inappropriate action against some component of the myelin sheath.

As a result of the alteration in the blood–brain barrier, immunoactive T-lymphocytes penetrate into the brain parenchyma. For a very long time, investigators focused on the role of the T-cell in causing the inflammatory reaction, but it is now known that antibodies against myelin components play an equally crucial role in pathogenesis. Other immunoactive substances in serum, including complement, interferon-gamma, as well as B-lymphocytes and macrophages, also cross the now permeable blood–brain barrier and play a still unknown role in the attack on the oligodendroglial–myelin complex. The exact mechanism by which the myelin sheath is injured is unknown. Cytokines secreted by T-cells have been proposed as the agents of myelinoclasia. The role of the oligodendrocyte in the pathogenetic cascade also remains in dispute, and many claim that it is it, rather than the myelin sheath, that is the primary target of the process. Some neuropathologists have claimed the disintegration of myelin is secondary to the destruction of oligodendrocytes in early MS lesions, but others have shown that these cells are not affected until later, as victims of non-specific destruction.

The primary effects of MS are inflammation and edema. Myelin destruction does not necessarily follow. Spontaneous resolution of the inflammation and edema without destruction frequently occurs, and provides a logical explanation for the very short duration of some symptoms. Remyelination occurs even in the earliest lesions, but is generally relatively inefficient and much too slow to account for clin-

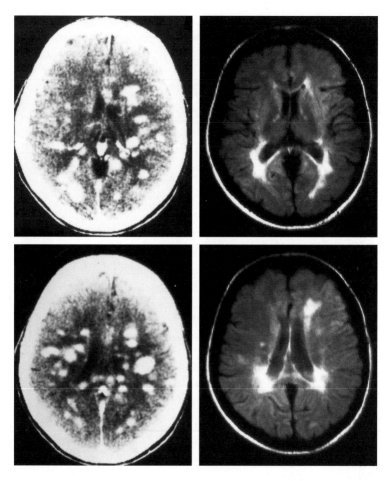

Figure 8 Double-dose (iodinated contrast) delayed CT scans (left) of a 32-year-old multiple sclerosis patient who experienced a severe exacerbation, show numerous areas of enhancement. The MRIs (right), obtained approximately 2 months later, after recovery, show few areas of increased signal intensity (AISI). With the possible exception of the enhanced area at the superior angle of the left ventricle, none of the areas of BBB alteration seen on CT are evident on MRI. Their disappearance so soon after clinical recovery suggests that the contrast enhancement represents edema rather than demyelination, as remyelination does not occur within such a short period of time. From Poser *et al.*, 1987; reproduced with permission of the American Society of Radiology

ical improvement within only a few days. Another explanation is the activation of alternative or supplementary physiological pathways.

After myelin is destroyed, it is replaced by a glial scar. It is such scars that have given MS its name. The destruction of myelin releases a number of its structural components, including cholesterol, fatty acids, myelin basic protein, myelin-associated glycoprotein, myelin-oligodendrocyte glycoprotein, proteolipid protein, phospholipids, cerebrosides, sphingomyelin and gangliosides. These substances may enter the bloodstream via the permeable blood–brain barrier and, in turn, provoke an immune response from systemic lymphocytes, thereby causing a vicious circle that results in a self-perpetuating condition. This may also be a possible explanation for the intermittent progression of the disease. Serial MRI studies with gadolinium enhancement have shown that the blood–brain barrier may remain permeable for an indefinite period of time.

Longitudinal imaging and evoked response studies have shown that the disease is relentlessly progressive, even in the absence of clinical exacerbations. This may be better understood if the disease is described as comparable to volcanic island chains, such as Hawaii, where only the tip of the undersea volcanoes are apparent, but with activity continuing unseen beneath the surface of the ocean (Figure 9). It is postulated that, in MS, periods of immune activity, probably stimulated by non-specific viral infections, alternate with periods of immunoquiescence.

The current status of our understanding – or lack thereof – of the role of the immune system in MS has been thus summarized by Cedric Raine as follows:

'In sum, while no single immune system molecule can be assigned as unusual to the CSF of MS, and, while there appears to be nothing unique about the manner in which the CNS responds to inflammation, the true uniqueness of the situation in MS is probably related to the many normally sequestered, specific antigens within the myelin sheath and the biology of the myelinating cell, the oligodendrocyte.'

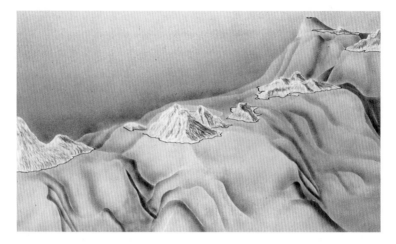

Figure 9 The disease process in multiple sclerosis can be compared with volcanic island chains such as the Hawaiian Islands, where only the tips of the volcanic structures protrude above sea level while unseen activity continues below

Pathology

Because MS is a disease of the myelin sheath, lesions are mostly found in white matter, but, because myelinated fibers are present in gray masses, lesions may be seen in gray matter as well. On gross sections of the brain, plaques appear as yellowish, slightly shrunken areas that are dense glial scars (Figures 10 and 11).

An important characteristic of MS lesions, as seen by various myelin sheath stains, is their very well-defined edge, described as looking as if they have been 'cut out with a cookie cutter' (Figures 12–14). This clearly differentiates the lesions of MS from those of acute disseminated encephalomyelitis. Inflammatory reactions, consisting mostly of lymphocytes and edema, are usually noted around the small blood vessels, especially in acute cases. Variable amounts of fat-staining lipid material, the so-called myelin abbau, can be observed in macrophages along with myelin fragments (Figures 15 and 16). The intensity of the fat staining is a good index of the age of the lesion: younger lesions contain greater amounts of lipid. Large abnormal astrocytes, termed 'gemistocytic astrocytes', are often seen at the sites of lesions (Figure 17) and may form large masses mimicking astrocytic tumors, leading to misinterpretation on biopsy. Classical MS lesions are periaxile in that the axon appears unaffected even when the myelin sheath has completely disintegrated. In older, more severe lesions, however, the axon is atrophic or has disappeared entirely. Necrosis may be seen, especially in acute lesions. Although axonal, and even neuronal, involvement was known to occur in MS for 100 years, the extent and significance of the damage were seriously underestimated until recently. It is now believed that the destruction of axons accounts for most clinical disability.

MS lesions vary considerably in size, ranging from only a few millimeters to plaques involving almost the entire centrum semiovale. Asymmetry is the rule and no part of the CNS is spared. Lesions are frequently noted in the spinal cord, especially the cervical portion, as well as, classically, the brain stem and cerebellum, and the cerebral

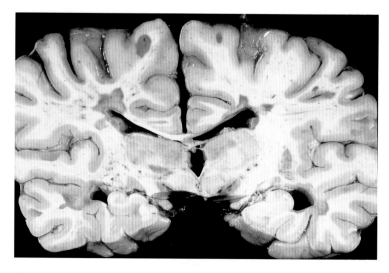

Figure 10 Unstained gross coronal sections of brain. Note the typical dark-colored periventricular and parenchymatous lesions

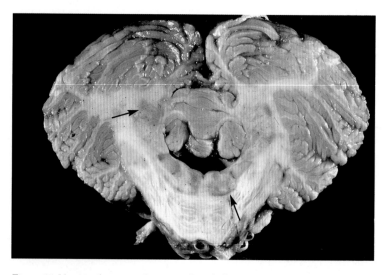

Figure 11 Unstained gross axial section of cerebellum. Note the typical involvement of the dentate nuclei and periventricular lesions (arrows)

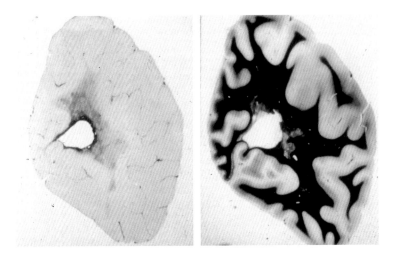

Figure 12 Celloidin sections of occipital lobe showing several small periventricular areas of demyelination. Nissl staining (left) shows reactive gliosis extending well beyond the plaques; Weigert staining (right) shows pale-staining, relatively restricted, demyelination. Courtesy of Professor H. Shiraki, University of Tokyo, Japan

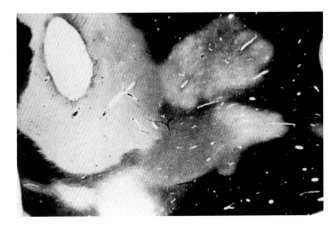

Figure 13 Celloidin section showing different intensities of staining. There is total loss of myelin in some plaques, represented by the absence of color, whereas, in other plaques, there is only pallor of the myelin. These 'shadow' plaques are believed by some to represent remyelination. Courtesy of Professor H. Shiraki, University of Tokyo, Japan

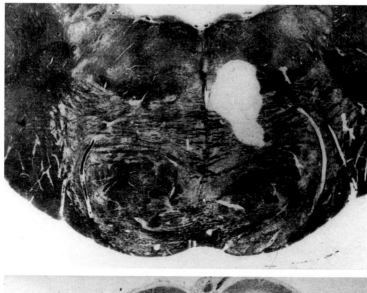

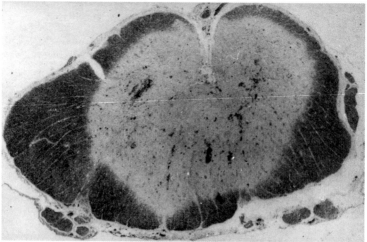

Figure 14 Weigert staining reveals a well-delineated multiple sclerosis plaque in the pons (upper) and a large plaque involving nearly the entire section of the cervical spinal cord (lower). The patient was a black Senegalese. Courtesy of Professor Michel Dumas, Institute of Neurological Epidemiology and Tropical Neurology, Limoges, France

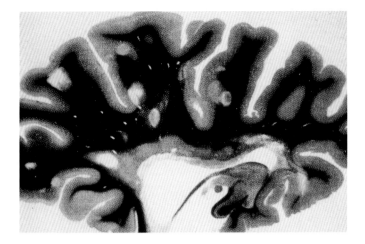

Figure 15 Celloidin section of brain shows that the age of multiple sclerosis lesions can be gauged from the color intensity of the stained fat, representing the abbau products of myelinoclasia: the redder the fat, the younger the lesion. Abbau products are no longer present in old lesions. Combined myelin–fat stains. From Roizin *et al.*, 1946; reproduced with permission of Williams and Wilkins

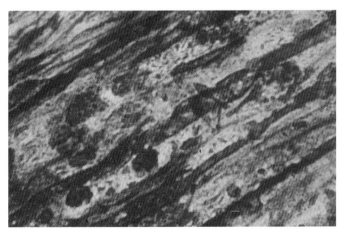

Figure 16 Histology (high-powered view of the same section as in Figure 15) shows fat-containing macrophages (arrow) scattered among degenerating myelin sheaths. Combined myelin–fat stains. From Roizin *et al.*, 1946; reproduced with permission of Williams and Wilkins

29

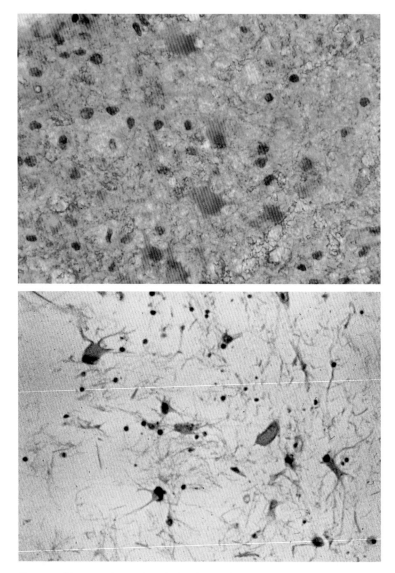

Figure 17 Histology of an early multiple sclerosis plaque shows gemistocytic astrocytes, seen with H&E–Luxol fast blue (upper) and Golgi (lower) staining

hemispheres. The optic nerves and optic chiasm are frequently involved. The median longitudinal fasciculus is eventually affected in many cases, causing the almost pathognomonic internuclear ophthalmoplegia. The basal ganglia, thalamus and hypothalamus, and dentate nuclei may also be sites of lesions. In exceptional circumstances, peripheral nerves may become involved. In regard to cranial nerves, lesions of the sensory nuclei of the trigeminal nerve, the intraparenchymal portion of the facial nerve and connections of the acoustic nerves are not uncommonly encountered. Tic douloureux, or trigeminal neuralgia, in a subject of less than 40 years of age, is virtually pathognomonic of MS.

Certain unusual forms of MS have been recognized, mostly on the basis of their pathological appearance. Balo's disease is characterized by the presence of concentric bands of normal-looking myelin alternating with areas of demyelination (Figures 18 and 19). These areas may be relatively large and may occupy a good part of the centrum semiovale. The clinical course of Balo's disease is usually one of rapid progression. However, similar areas of concentric alternating demyelination have been seen in otherwise unremarkable cases of MS and in acute disseminated encephalomyelitis. Another variant of MS is diffuse sclerosis, or Schilder's disease. True Schilder's disease is extremely rare, and is defined as the presence of very large bilateral, slightly asymmetrical areas of demyelination in the cerebral white matter (Figures 20 and 21). Diffuse sclerosis is usually seen in children. The very large lesions are often associated with the more typical small disseminated lesions of MS. The nosological situation of what is often designated as a variant of MS – Devic's disease or neuromyelitis optica – is the subject of dispute. Lesions affect only the optic nerves and spinal cord, not necessarily simultaneously. It is estimated that only approximately one-quarter of cases of neuromyelitis optica are cases of MS; the rest are most probably instances of postinfectious encephalomyelitis.

Electron microscopy of the classical lesion of MS reveals a number of characteristic changes (Figure 22). One of the earliest changes is separation of the myelin lamellae by edema. This is often followed by the appearance of macrophages containing myelin debris or fragments, abrupt tapering of the myelin sheath, and axonal denudation. Evidence of remyelination may be seen even in the earliest lesions.

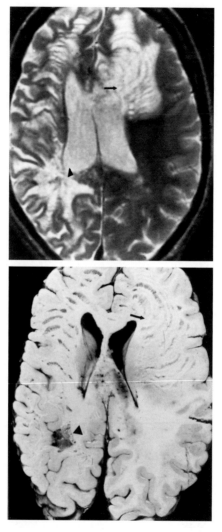

Figure 18 Axial MRI (upper) and gross appearance (lower) of brain in Baló's disease. There is concentric demyelination (arrows) and another lesion (indicated by the triangles). Courtesy of Dr George Collins, State University of New York at Syracuse, from Gharagozloo *et al.*, 1994; reproduced with permission of the Radiological Society of America

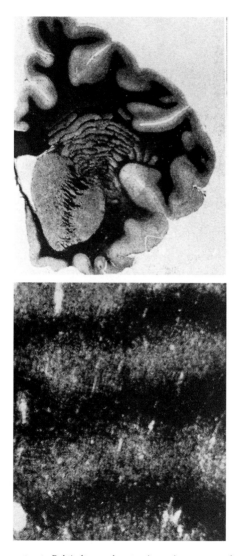

Figure 19 Brain section in Baló's disease showing (upper) concentric demyelination in the right centrum semiovale. High-power view of the same area (lower) shows alternating bands of normal myelin and remyelination. Weigert stains. Courtesy of Professor H. Shiraki, University of Tokyo, Japan

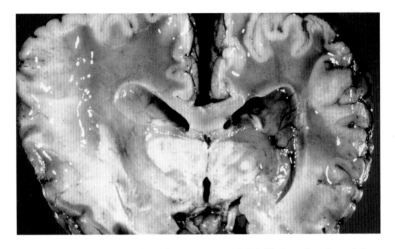

Figure 20 Gross specimen of brain from a patient with Schilder's myelinoclastic diffuse sclerosis shows large bilateral areas of demyelination

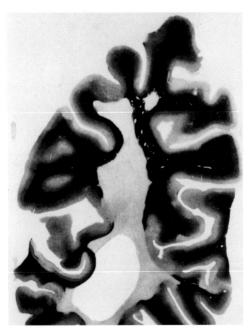

Figure 21 Celloidin section of brain from a patient with Schilder's myelinoclastic diffuse sclerosis shows a large plaque occupying most of the centrum semiovale. Weigert stain. Courtesy of Professor H. Shiraki, University of Tokyo, Japan

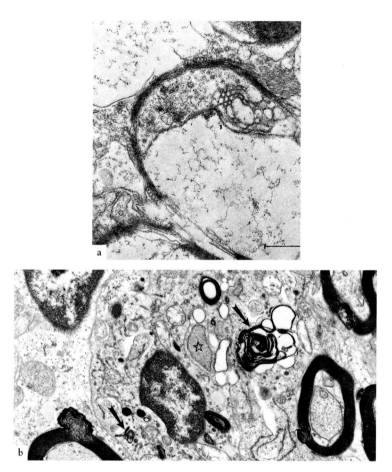

Figure 22 a–h Electron micrographs showing (a) vesicular dissolution of myelin in acute multiple sclerosis (bar = 0.5 μm); (b) a naked axon (indicated by star) enveloped by a macrophage containing fragments of undegraded (native periodicity) myelin debris (arrows), indicative of recent uptake (bar = 1.0 μm)
Selected by Professor Ingrid Allen and Dr John Kirk, Queen's University of Belfast and the Royal Victoria Hospital, Belfast, Northern Ireland. Courtesy of Dr John Kirk (a, b), with permission of Blackwell Science (a); from Allen, 1991, with permission of Churchill Livingstone (b) (*continued*)

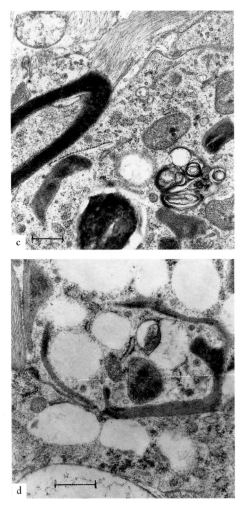

Figure 22 *Continued* Electron micrographs showing (c) various stages of myelin degradation in a macrophage (bar = 1.0 μm); (d) lyre bodies and lipid droplets in a macrophage (bar = 0.5 μm)
Selected by Professor Ingrid Allen and Dr John Kirk, Queen's University of Belfast and the Royal Victoria Hospital, Belfast, Northern Ireland. Courtesy of Dr Michael Hutchinson (c, d); from Allen and Kirk. 1992, with permission of Edward Arnold (c, d) (*continued*)

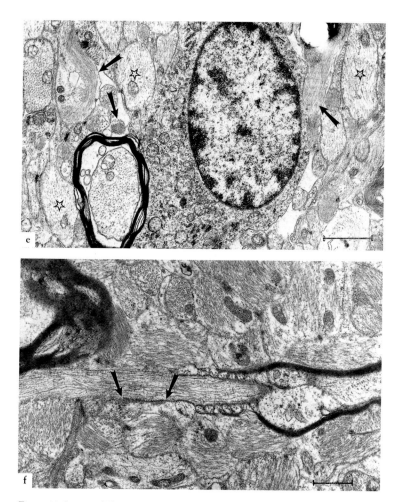

Figure 22 *Continued* Electron micrographs showing (e) an isolated oligodendrocyte and myelin sheath among naked axons (indicated by stars) and astrocytic processes (arrows; bar = 20 μm); (f) periaxial segmental demyelination, in which loss of myelin internodal segment has resulted in paranodal axolemmal specialization (between arrows). Filament-rich astrocytic processes surround the naked axon (bar = 2.0 μm).

Selected by Professor Ingrid Allen and Dr John Kirk, Queen's University of Belfast and the Royal Victoria Hospital, Belfast, Northern Ireland. Courtesy of Dr John Kirk (e, f); from Allen, 1991, with permission of Churchill Livingstone (e) (*continued*)

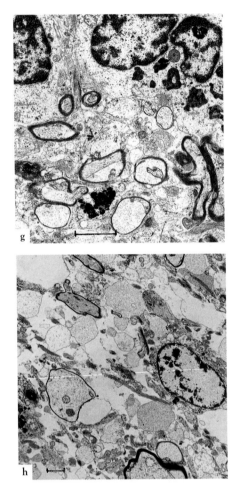

Figure 24 *Continued* Electron micrographs showing (g) subcortical white matter from an area of reduced myelin density at the edge of a plaque. Many of the axons show abnormally thin (?remyelinated) myelin sheaths; macrophages are numerous but do not contain recent (normal periodicity) myelin debris. Astrocytic gliosis is pronounced (bar = 2.0 μm); (h) a large periventricular plaque in which naked axons persist alongside thin remyelinated axons and fine astrocytic processes containing bundled filaments (bar = 2.0 μm)

Selected by Professor Ingrid Allen and Dr John Kirk, Queen's University of Belfast and the Royal Victoria Hospital, Belfast, Northern Ireland. Courtesy of Dr John Kirk (g, h)

Physiology

Normal motor and sensory function is dependent upon the rapid propagation of the nerve impulse along myelinated nerve fibers; this time is measured in milliseconds. The myelin sheath is interrupted at regular intervals by nodes of Ranvier, where the axon is denuded. Because the axon has a high resistance to the electrical impulse and the speed of conduction is too slow, there is an alternative mechanism called 'saltatory conduction'. This is where the electrical impulse jumps from one node of Ranvier to the next, while achieving the required conduction velocity. However, if the distance between the available nodes is too great because of destruction of myelin segments, the impulse cannot bridge the gap and saltatory conduction is either impaired or abolished. The electrical impulse must then travel via the slow axonal route.

Signs and symptoms may appear in some MS patients due to slowing of nerve conduction caused by a rise in body temperature as a result of either ambient heat or fever (Uhthoff's phenomenon). The latter is a common cause of pseudo-exacerbations. A body temperature increase of as little as 0.1°C may be sufficient to cause such signs and symptoms, which disappear upon cooling. By far the most common cause of these pseudo-exacerbations is an unsuspected urinary tract infection.

Clinical aspects

Multiple sclerosis most frequently affects the optic nerve and chiasm, brain stem, cerebellum and the cervical spinal cord. The presence of spondylosis often contributes to the formation of plaques in that region. This preferential involvement determines the frequency of the signs and symptoms observed in MS patients (Table 1). Because it is often difficult, especially on the basis of patient history, to separate symptoms from signs, the clinical features listed in Table 1 are presented as symptom/sign combinations.

Determination of the exact clinical onset of the disease is important for epidemiological investigations. Often, non-specific symptoms such as headache, seizure, dizziness or back pain are mentioned as the first clinical manifestations of the illness. These onset symptoms of MS may be divided into those which are 'definite' and those which are 'possible'. These symptoms must last for at least 24 hours.

The definite symptoms include unilateral optic/retrobulbar monocular color blindness, oscillopsia, transient scanning speech, transverse myelitis, Lhermitte's symptom, gait ataxia, unilateral dysmetria/intention tremor/incoordination, sensory useless hand syndrome, and transient weakness/paresthesias of the entire limb. The following are also considered to be definite, but only if the patient is less than 40 years of age: tic douloureux, hemifacial spasm, acute unilateral diminution of hearing, transient acute non-positional vertigo, transient painless urinary retention, and transient painless urinary urgency or incontinence in men.

For the following possible symptoms to be considered markers of MS onset, they must be followed by a definite symptom within 2 years: unilateral facial palsy, organic erectile dysfunction, and painful tonic spasms. Transient painless urinary frequency in men, and transient hemiparesis are acceptable only in patients under age 40.

Table 1 Initial symptoms, clinical course and predominant clinical category in 461 MS patients (From Paty and Poser, 1984, reproduced with permission). Data are given as the number (%) of patients

	Frequency		
	Women (n = 279)	Men (n = 182)	Total (n = 461)
Symptom			
Visual loss in one eye	54 (18)	24 (13)	78 (17)
Double vision	27 (10)	35 (19)	62 (13)
Disturbance of balance and gait	38 (14)	45 (25)	83 (18)
Sensory disturbance in limbs	72 (26)	79 (43)	151 (33)
Sensory disturbance in face	10 (4)	6 (3)	16 (3)
Acute myelitic syndrome	20 (7)	6 (3)	26 (6)
Lhermitte's symptom	7 (3)	6 (3)	13 (3)
Pain	5 (2)	3 (2)	8 (2)
Progressive weakness	27 (9)	18 (8)	45 (10)
Clinical course			
Relapsing and remitting	164 (59)	93 (51)	257 (56)
Chronic progressive	67 (24)	60 (33)	127 (28)
Combined	66 (24)	29 (16)	55 (12)
Benign	39 (14)	16 (9)	55 (12)
Predominant clinical category			
Spinal	128 (46)	134 (74)	262 (57)
Cerebellar	23 (8)	35 (19)	58 (13)
Cerebral	11(4)	7 (4)	18 (4)

Clinical course

The course of MS is usually classified as:

(1) Classic relapsing and remitting type (RRMS), which represents about one-third of the cases;

(2) Primary progressive (PPMS), which is uncommon and represents about 10% of cases; and

(3) Secondary progressive (SPMS), which follows a relapsing–remitting course.

'Burned-out' cases are rarely mentioned, yet constitute approximately 20% of cases. In such a case, the disease seems to have become arrested. Most of these patients have become wheelchair-bound, but their upper extremities remain functional.

MS can also follow a hyperacute course, leading to death in a matter of a few weeks; this type has been called 'Marburg disease'. Many of those cases are actually cases of acute monophasic disseminated encephalomyelitis rather than MS.

It is frequently suggested that these various clinical categories represent separate disease entities, but it is more logical and correct to consider that they are simply the phenotypic responses to a single disease of individuals with different genetic endowment and immunologic history. In every one of these clinical groups, the end result of the disease process is the same, the sharp-edged plaque.

Exacerbations of MS often follow on the heels of a viral infection. Because such infections may be very mild or even clinically silent, the triggering event may not be recognized. The role of trauma, electrical injury, vaccinations and emotional stress in precipitating attacks of MS, although relevant, remains controversial.

The correlation between the number, site and size of MS lesions, as revealed by neuroimaging and at autopsy, and clinical manifestations is poor. Many plaques involve the so-called 'silent' areas of the brain. The reason why some lesions do not cause neurological dysfunction is best explained by the theoretical concept of the 'safety factor'. The disease process must impair conduction in a critical, minimum number of fibers of motor or sensory tracts before clinical dysfunction occurs. The number of available fibers above this minimum number constitutes the safety factor. If the signs and symptoms are due only to inflammation and edema, they will be reversible. When the safety factor is totally abolished by myelinoclasia, the patient will have permanent signs or symptoms (Figure 23).

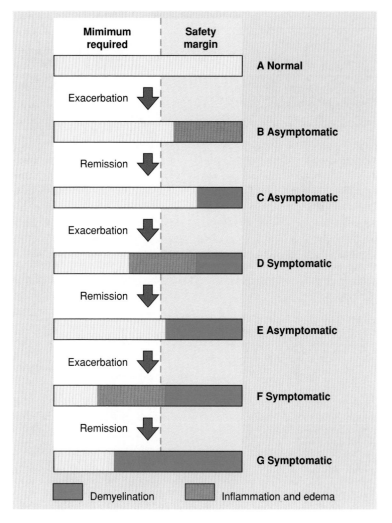

Figure 23 Safety factor in the progression of multiple sclerosis: as long as the required minimum number of nerve fibers remains intact, the patient is asymptomatic. When symptomatic myelin edema occurs during an exacerbation, remission may result in either complete or partial recovery, depending upon functional restoration of the required number of fibers, or in a permanent deficit, as a result of myelinoclasia. From Poser, 1993; reproduced with permission of Elsevier Science BV

Diagnosis

Diagnostic criteria

The diagnosis of MS is a clinical exercise based on the characteristic dissemination of the lesions in both space and time. This principle applies to the overwhelming majority of cases. Until recently, the diagnostic criteria that have been virtually universally adopted were those first published in 1983. New criteria (McDonald *et al.* 2001) have now been published and are becoming widely accepted. They will be discussed later. Because they emphasize MRI, which is not readily available in many parts of the world, a simplified version of the 1983 scheme is reproduced in Table 2.

The following explanatory comments are an integral part of the scheme:

Attack (bout, episode, exacerbation): must last at least 24 hours

Paraclinical evidence: demonstration by neuroimaging (CT or MRI) or evoked potential studies of CNS lesions that may or may not

Table 2 Diagnostic criteria for multiple sclerosis (From Poser *et al.*, 1983, with permission)

Category	Attack	Clinical evidence	Paraclinical evidence	CSF oligoclonal bands or increasing IgG
Clinical definite				
1	2	2		
2	2	1 and	1	
Laboratory definite				
1	2	1 or	1	+
2	1	2		+
3	1	1 and	1	+
+, present				

previously have caused signs or symptoms. Such lesions must be at locations different from those recorded by history or examination

Remission: a definite improvement, lasting for at least a month

Laboratory support: this applies only to the examination of CSF for an increased level of immunoglobulin G (IgG) and the presence of oligoclonal bands (see CSF below)

The new MS diagnostic criteria of McDonald

The explosion in the availability and use of MRI has made almost mandatory the inclusion of imaging criteria. The new scheme is reproduced in Table 3.

Patients are divided into three groups: MS, non-MS and possible. It is somewhat difficult to appreciate why the last category was included. For the first time, primary progressive MS (PPMS) is carefully characterized, the problem of pseudo-exacerbations is mentioned, and the diagnostic value of brain stem auditory and somatosensory evoked potentials is questioned. Symptoms are not acceptable. Regarding MRI, the criteria lack a qualitative dimension which is so important in distinguishing between MS and disseminated encephalomyelitis, but those for spinal cord lesions and for dissemination in time are most useful.

Optic fundus and visual fields

Because the optic nerve and the visual system are so frequently involved, and the optic nerve head is the only externally visible part of the CNS, examining the optic fundus and plotting the visual fields provide valuable clinical information (Figures 24 and 25).

Table 3 McDonald diagnostic criteria (after McDonald *et al.* 2001)

Clinical presentation	Additional data needed for diagnosis of MS
• Two or more attacks *and* • Objective clinical evidence of two or more lesions	• None
• Two or more attacks *and* • Objective clinical evidence of one lesion	• Dissemination in space on MRI; or two or more lesions consistent with MS and positive CSF *or* • Await clinical attack implicating a different site
• One attack *and* • Objective clinical evidence of two or more lesions	• Dissemination in time on MRI *or* • Second clinical attack
• One attack *and* • Objective clinical evidence of one lesion	1. Dissemination in space on MRI; or positive CSF with two or more lesions on MRI consistent with MS *and* 2. Dissemination in time on MRI; or second clinical attack
• Insidious neurological	1. Positive CSF progression *and* 2. Dissemination in space by MRI with nine or more T2 lesions, *or* two or more lesions in spinal cord, *or* four to eight brain lesions + one spinal cord lesion, *or* abnormal VEP with four to eight brain lesions *or* < four brain lesions + one spinal cord lesion with abnormal VEP *and* 3. Dissemination in time on MRI or continued progression for 1 year

CSF = cerebrospinal fluid; VEP = visual evoked potentials

Confirmatory laboratory procedures

The following comments apply to both sets of diagnostic criteria. With few exceptions, the laboratory procedures described below should be used only if the clinical information and findings on neurological examination are insufficient to warrant making the diagnosis of definite MS. Thus, these procedures are intended to confirm a suspicion of MS or, on rare occasions, rule out conditions such as disseminated encephalomyelitis (in particular, the recurrent and multiphasic types), Lyme disease, HTLV-I-associated paraparesis, sarcoidosis, etc. *Contrary to widely held opinion, an MRI or a lumbar puncture is not necessary to make the diagnosis of MS.*

Examination of cerebrospinal fluid

Lumbar puncture as an adjunct for the diagnosis of MS has become increasingly rare, but remains an essential procedure when other conditions, such as Lyme disease, sarcoidosis, HTLV-I-associated paraparesis, AIDS, and neurosyphilis, must be ruled out. Thus, it remains a useful confirmatory test for MS.

In an acute attack of MS, there is often a slight elevation of lymphocytes and of total protein. A CSF protein level greater than 75 mg/100 ml should raise serious doubts about the diagnosis of MS.

Measurement of the level of IgG is an important part of the CSF examination. The simplest and most reliable measurement is the percentage of total protein: >15% is considered abnormal. However, an elevated CSF IgG is non-specific. It is often observed in many other conditions affecting the nervous system. A more useful examination is the search for oligoclonal bands in the gammaglobulin fraction of protein (Figures 26 and 27). To be significant, there must be at least two bands

Footnote to Table 3: Positive CSF = presence of oligoclonal IgG bands different from any such bands in serum and/or presence of an elevated IgG index. Abnormal VEP can be used to supplement information provided by the clinical examination to give objective evidence of a second lesion (provided the only clinically expressed lesion did not affect the visual pathways). Other types of evoked potentials were viewed as contributing little to the diagnosis of MS

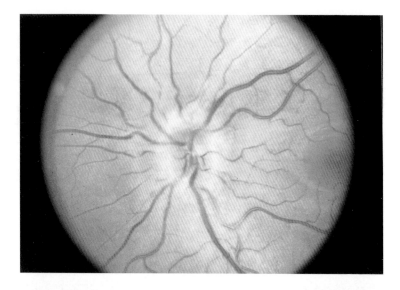

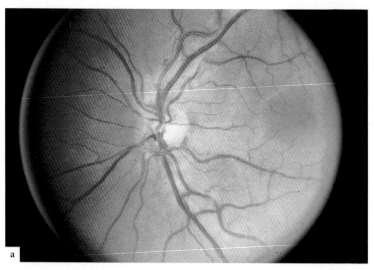

a

Figure 24 a–d Funduscopy in multiple sclerosis showing (a) papillitis (upper) vs a normal fundus (lower). Courtesy of Dr Simmons Lessell, Massachusetts Eye and Ear Infirmary, Boston, MA (*continued*)

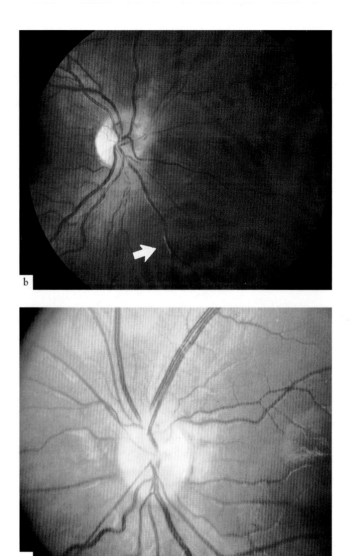

Figure 24 *Continued* Funduscopy in multiple sclerosis showing (b) mild segmental venous sheathing (arrow); (c) severe optic atrophy. Courtesy of Dr Jason Barton, Beth Israel Deaconess Medical Center, Boston, MA (*continued*)

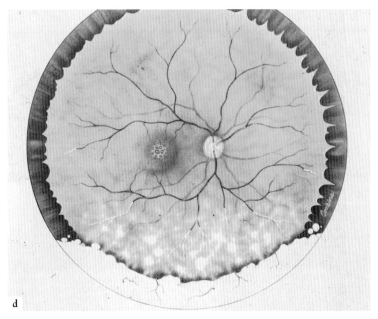

d

Figure 24 *Continued* (d) Pars planitis: watercolor of a flattened retina showing the optic disk and macula (towards the center) as well as the most anterior portion of the retina, the pars plana (scalloped yellow margin), which lies just behind the ciliary body. Periphlebitis is evident in some of the distal portions of the retinal veins. Inflammatory cells in the vitreous have settled over the inferior retina, giving the appearance of 'snowbanks'. Severe cases may also have cystoid macular edema, as shown here.
Courtesy of Drs Janet Davis, Bascom–Palmer Eye Institute, and Noble David, University of Miami, FL

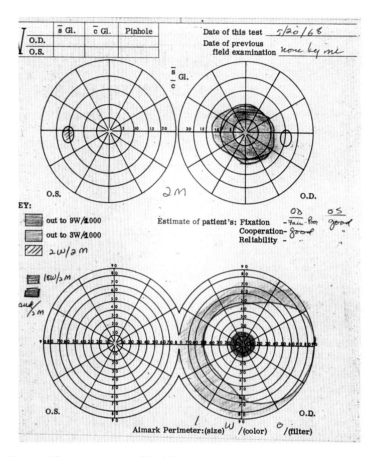

Figure 25 Tangent screen visual field showing a central scotoma due to optic atrophy subsequent to optic neuritis. Courtesy of Dr Simmons Lessell, Massachusetts Eye and Ear Infirmary, Boston, MA

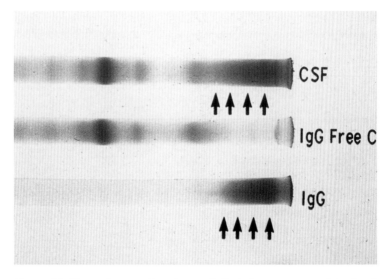

Figure 26 Electrophoresis of cerebrospinal fluid showing increased levels of immunoglobulin G (arrows), a non-specific finding

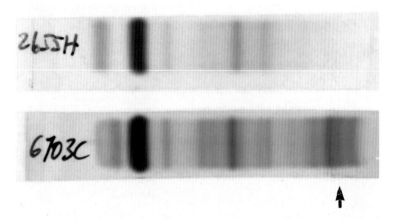

Figure 27 Electrophoresis of cerebrospinal fluid showing (upper) normal vs (lower) x80 increased concentration; three oligoclonal bands can be seen in the IgG fraction (arrow). Coomassie brilliant blue stain. Courtesy of Dr James Faix, Beth Israel Deaconess Medical Center, Boston, MA

present and none in the serum. The presence of oligoclonal bands in the CSF is not specific for MS; they may be noted in other conditions. They never disappear from the CSF in MS, but may do so in disseminated encephalomyelitis.

Evoked potential studies

Pattern-reversal visual evoked responses are particularly useful in identifying optic nerve and chiasmatic lesions in patients who have had no symptoms or signs of involvement of the visual system, because they may be delayed in 75% of such patients, including those with normal visual acuity. The critical measurement is that of the peak, designated as P100 (Figure 28). The amplitude of the response is of little portent. Interocular differences in P100 delay are usually meaningless. Because

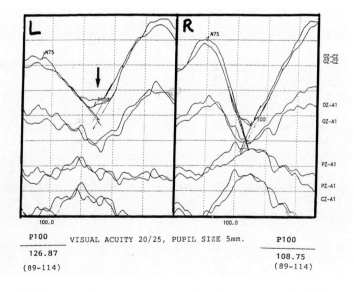

Figure 28 Visual evoked response in a patient with left optic atrophy. The P100 wave on the left is delayed compared with that on the right. Courtesy of Dr Frank Drislane, Beth Israel Deaconess Medical Center, Boston, MA

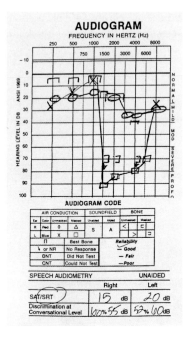

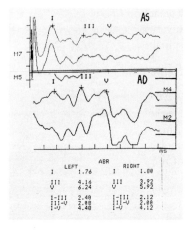

Figure 29 Audiogram (upper) showing acute partial hearing loss in left ear, specifically, hearing loss at high frequencies; (lower) the brain stem auditory evoked response shows delay of waves ll and V in the left ear. Courtesy of Dr Carl Lieberman, Framingham, MA

the response is modified by changes in visual acuity, it is imperative that the patient wears prescribed corrective lenses during the test. Delay in P100 is far from specific for MS lesions of the optic system; in addition to poor fixation and changes in visual acuity, many other conditions may give false-positive results. Among the more common ones are glaucoma, alcohol ingestion, cerebrovascular disease, spinocerebellar degeneration, all types of optic atrophy, and the use of many commonly prescribed drugs.

Brain-stem auditory responses are much less useful because they are positive in only a small percentage of cases, even in the presence of overt clinical signs of brain-stem involvement, such as internuclear ophthalmoplegia. In patients with MS, the most frequently observed delay is between waves III and V (Figure 29). Peripheral delays simply indicate acoustic nerve lesions, which are usually unrelated to MS.

Somatosensory evoked responses are rarely of value and are almost invariably and needlessly performed in patients who clearly have spinal cord lesions. They are often painful.

Neuroimaging

Computed tomography

Despite the general availability of MRI in most countries, computed tomography (CT) scanning will undoubtedly remain, for many years to come, the only neuroimaging procedure available in the poorer areas of the world. Although CT resolution is far below that of MRI, the cost of the equipment is only a fraction of the cost of the latter (Figures 30–32). Doubling, or even tripling, the dose of intravenous iodinated

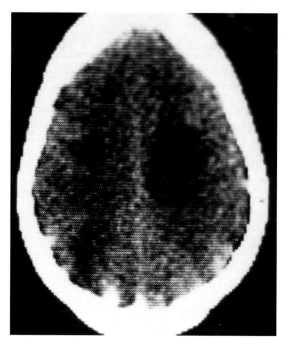

Figure 30 Axial CT scan of a multiple sclerosis patient with an acute left hemiparesis showing a large area of hypodensity in the right hemisphere, and two smaller areas in the left

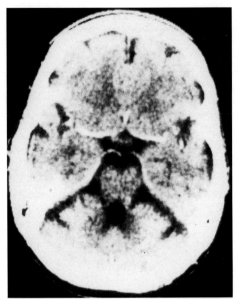

Figure 31 Axial CT scan showing severe brain stem and cerebellar atrophy

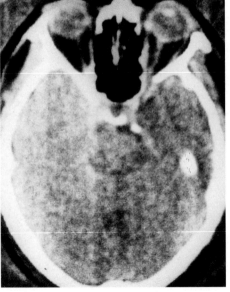

Figure 32 Axial CT scan showing bilateral optic atrophy

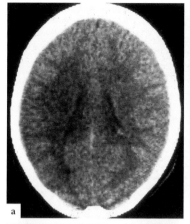

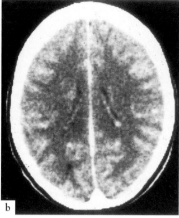

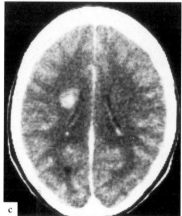

Figure 33 Axial CT scans, using iodinated contrast and taken after a 60-min delay, compare the effects of (a) no contrast with (b) 300 mg and (c) 600 mg of contrast. With 300 mg, the left posterior frontal lesion is only faintly seen whereas doubling the dose renders the lesion much more obvious. Courtesy of Drs Fernando Vinuela and George Ebers, University of Western Ontario, London, Canada

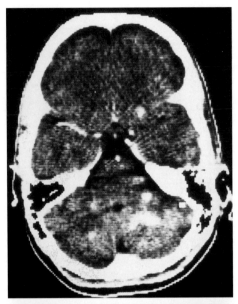

Figure 34 Double-dose contrast delayed axial CT scan shows multiple lesions in the cerebellum

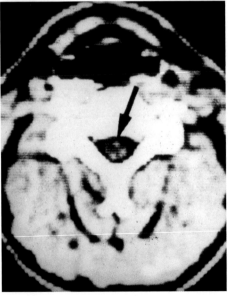

Figure 35 Axial CT scan, using iodinated contrast, shows lesions (arrows) at the level of C4 of the spinal cord. Plaques of the spinal cord are rarely seen by CT

contrast medium and delaying imaging for one or two hours have greatly enhanced the ability of CT to reveal MS lesions, even in the spinal cord (Figures 33–35).

Magnetic resonance imaging

The introduction of magnetic resonance imaging (MRI) has completely revolutionized the diagnostic process of MS, but has proved to be a mixed blessing. The proliferation of MRI machines has led to their overuse and to misinterpretation of the images. At present, too often the diagnosis of MS has been based exclusively on the presence of areas of increased signal intensity (AISIs), which are most often referred to as 'lesions', visualized in the white matter on T2-weighted MRI scans (Figure 36).

Approximately 5–15% of clinically definite MS patients have completely normal MRIs on repeated examination. Conversely, there are patients with insignificant complaints who have MRI abnormalities that are similar to those frequently seen in symptomatic MS patients (Figures 37–39). The correlation between the number, site and size of MRI white matter AISIs and the clinical signs and symptoms of MS is very poor and unreliable. The often-used term 'burden of disease', based on the number and size of 'lesions', is misleading, as very large AISIs may be seen which have persisted for years in clinically normal subjects.

Attempts to establish reliable MRI diagnostic criteria have largely been unsuccessful, because the pattern and characteristics of images associated with MS are also seen in many other diseases. There are no MRI patterns of 'lesions', including the ovoid periventricular lesion, which are essential or even diagnostic of MS. The ones included in the McDonald et al. (2001) criteria were derived retrospectively from the images of patients who had had a clinically isolated syndrome who then had a second episode and thus were deemed to have MS.

A very important, but rarely emphasized, use of MRI is in the routine visualization of the cervical cord. In a surprisingly large number of MS patients, cervical cord plaques can be seen adjacent to areas of compression – whether actual, potential or intermittent – by spondylosis and/or herniated disks (Figures 40–42). It is possible that pressure from such extrinsic lesions may aggravate the underlying MS in addition to the myelopathic effects they produce. Obtaining lateral MRI views of the neck in flexion may reveal effacement of the ventral subarachnoid space or even cord compression that is not evident with the neck in a normal position, in particular in patients who have a neck injury.

Gadolinium enhancement of MRI has limited clinical application. Its routine clinical use is inappropriate and needlessly expensive. It is unusual to find an enhancing lesion that is not visible on the T2-weighted image (Figure 43). Treatment decisions of exacerbations

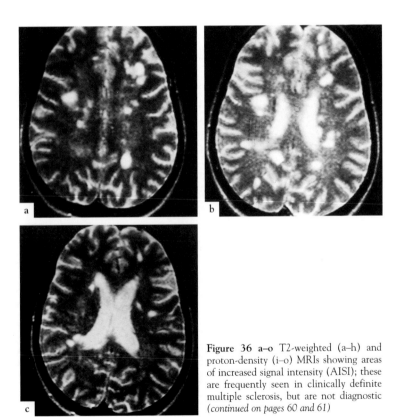

Figure 36 a–o T2-weighted (a–h) and proton-density (i–o) MRIs showing areas of increased signal intensity (AISI); these are frequently seen in clinically definite multiple sclerosis, but are not diagnostic *(continued on pages 60 and 61)*

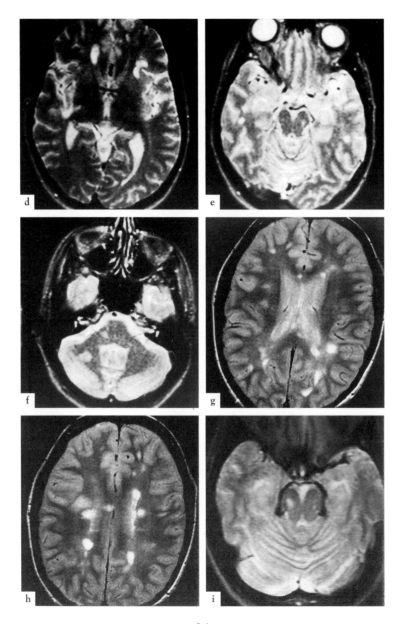

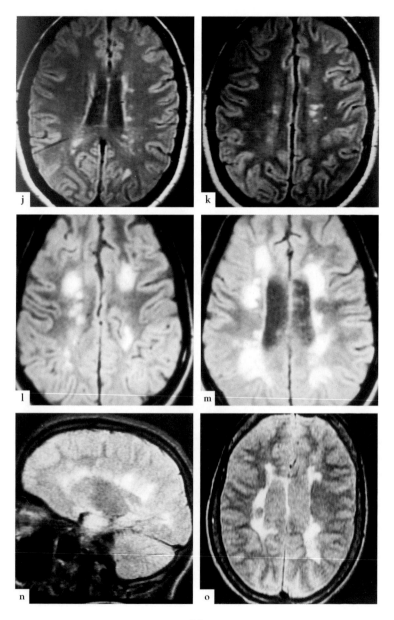

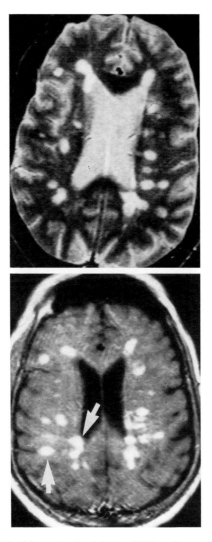

Figure 37 T2-weighted (upper) and gadolinium–EDTA-enhanced (lower) axial MRIs showing a number of ovoid lesions. Although many areas of increased signal intensity are seen on T2-weighting, other such areas (arrows) not revealed by T2-weighting are clearly seen with gadolinium–EDTA enhancement. This phenomenon is relatively uncommon

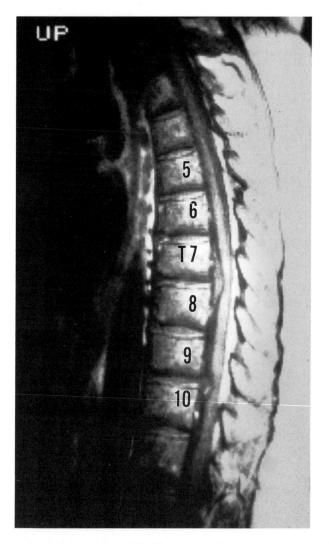

Figure 38 Sagittal proton density MRI of the spinal cord shows a completely extruded disk compressing the cord at the level of T7–8. Note the areas of increased signal intensity extending both above and below the site of compression. There is also cord compression at the T9–10 level. The patient had suffered from a fall around 2 months previously

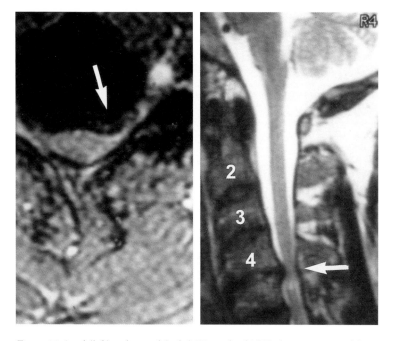

Figure 39 Axial (left) and sagittal (right) T2-weighted MRIs show severe spondylosis at C4–5 with cord compression. Note the areas of increased signal intensity immediately below the compression site (arrow; right). Spondylosis at C5–6 has obliterated the subarachnoid space anteriorly. The cord is shoved backwards, causing narrowing of the subarachnoid space posteriorly from C3–4 downwards. The axial view of C4–5 shows compression of the cord clearly

should be based on clinical considerations. At present, the reliability of evaluating long-term treatment by serial gadolinium-enhanced MRI has not been completely settled. While enhancement, which reflects the inflammatory reaction, and blood–brain barrier alteration, are often considered to be a sign of activity of the disease, its actuality is deceptive: blood–brain barrier alterations may have been present for 3 months or longer.

Variations in imaging protocols can help to distinguish separate components of the underlying pathological process (Figure 44). In addition

Figure 40 a–c Sagittal T2-weighted MRI taken 8 months after a whiplash injury to the neck shows loss of the normal cervical lordosis due to cervical muscle spasm (a). A posterior area of increased signal intensity is seen at the level of C3; another, larger and more dense, lies anterior to and below it. There is attenuation of the anterior subarachnoid space at C4–5, C5–6 and C6–7 levels. Sagittal T2-weighted MRIs taken 14 months later show less muscle spasm, and the area of increased signal intensity at C4 appears to

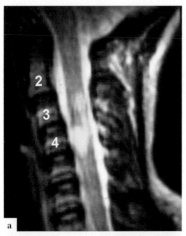

be less dense (b). There is attenuation of the subarachnoid space posteriorly at the level of C3 due to a fold in the ligament, which corresponds to the area of increased signal intensity at that level. With the neck in flexion (c), the anterior subarachoid space is markedly attenuated, especially at C4–5 and C5–6 levels, whereas the posterior space is greatly enlarged, presumably as a result of pressure on the cerebrospinal fluid surrounding the tethered cord. The posterior indentation at C3 persists. It is thought that violent hyperflexion of the neck at the time of whiplash injury was responsible for the formation of the C4 plaque. Courtesy of Dr Gerald O'Reilly, CHEM MRI, Stoneham, MA

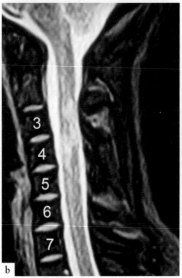

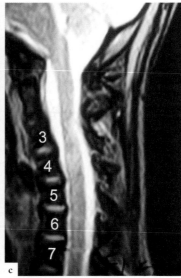

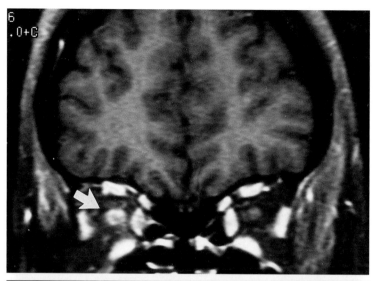

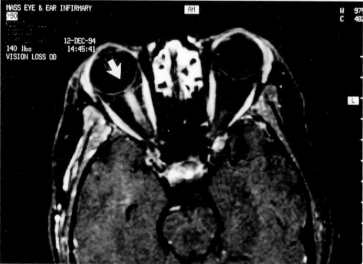

Figure 41 T2-weighted coronal (upper) and axial (lower) MRIs showing lesions resulting in right optic neuritis (arrows). Courtesy of Drs Simmons Lessell and Judith Warner, Massachusetts Eye and Ear Infirmary, Boston, MA

to inflammation, demyelination (magnetization transfer ratio), gliosis (T2-weighting reflecting increased water content), and axonal damage (reduction in diffusion tensor imaging anisotrophy and N-acetyl-aspartate spectra with chemical shift imaging, or the presence of 'black holes' with T1-weighting).

Imaging differential diagnoses

Many diseases of the nervous system that result in white-matter lesions seen by MRI are often erroneously diagnosed as MS. By far the most common of these is acute disseminated encephalomyelitis (ADEM) (Figure 45). However, the distribution and the size of the lesions in ADEM are quite characteristic and should rarely be confused with MS (Figures 46–48). Conversely, the AISIs may look the same as those often seen in MS. More difficult is the clinical differentiation of the

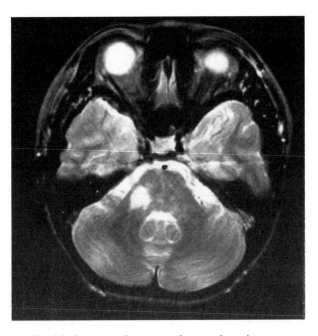

Figure 42 MRI of the brain stem shows areas of increased signal intensity in a patient with right facial palsy

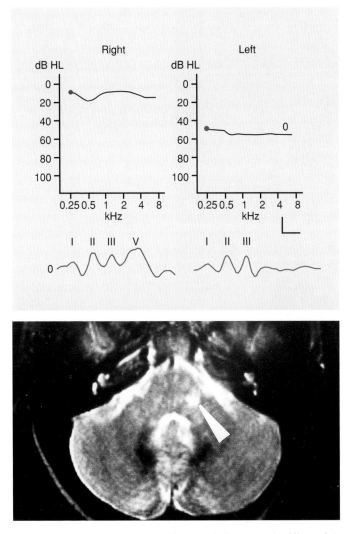

Figure 43 Audiogram (upper graphs), auditory evoked response (middle graphs) and MRI (lower) of a patient who had a sudden partial loss of hearing in the left ear. The audiogram shows decreased perception of all frequencies; the brain stem auditory evoked response shows absence of wave V; and the MRI shows areas of increased signal intensity in the left brain stem just above the superior olive (arrow)

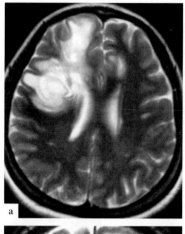

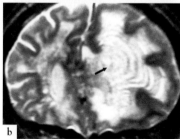

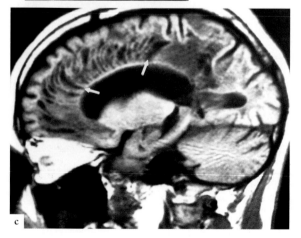

Figure 44 a–c MRI appearances of Balò's disease. Courtesy of Dr Chi-Jen Chen, Chang-Gung Medical College, Taipei, Taiwan, from Chen et al., 1996, reproduced with permission of Lippincott-Raven (a); and Dr George Collins, State University of New York at Syracuse, from Gharagozloo et al., 1994, reproduced with permission of the Radiological Society of America (b, c)

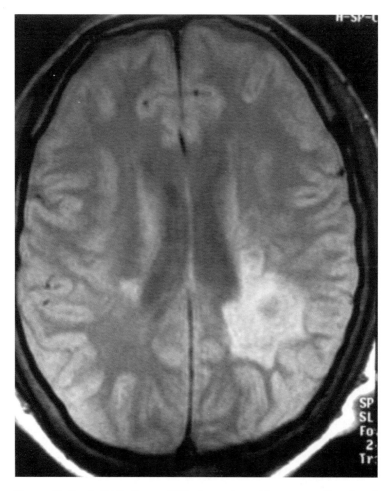

Figure 45 Pseudo-Baló's disease. MRI of a patient with recurrent disseminated encephalomyelitis. A number of similar cases have been erroneously published as examples of Baló's disease. Courtesy of Professor Vesna Brinar, University of Zagreb, Croatia

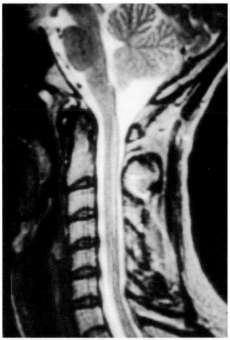

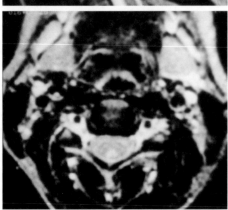

Figure 46 Sagittal (upper) and axial (lower) T2-weighted MRIs of a patient with ADEM showing a single, very long, area of increased signal intensity restricted to the posterior columns of the upper cervical cord. The patient's only complaint was clumsiness due to loss of positional sense in her hands

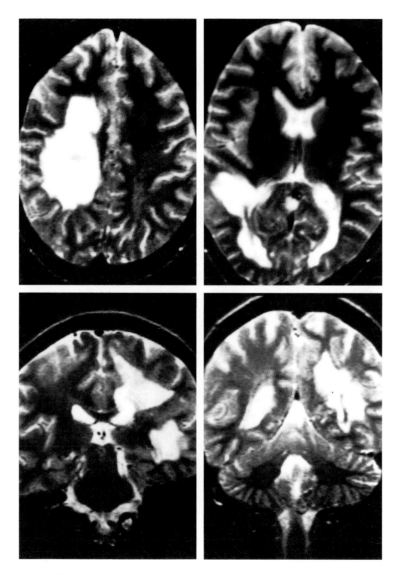

Figure 47 Coronal T2-weighted MRIs of a patient with postvaccination (influenza) encephalomyelitis

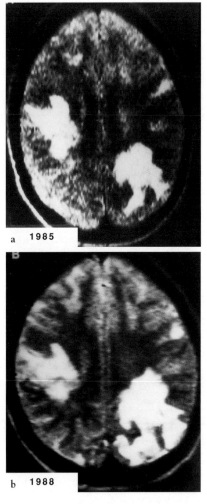

a 1985

b 1988

Figure 48 a and b Axial MRIs of ADEM in a 17-year-old girl who had a grand mal seizure accompanied by aphasia. Recovery was complete within 24 hours. MRI (a) showed enormous bilateral areas of increased signal intensity (AISI). The patient was asymptomatic for a year, until she had another seizure after discontinuing her anticonvulsant medication. Her neurological examination was normal, but MRI showed the same AISI. Three years later, the follow-up MRI (b) in this completely asymptomatic subject still showed the same AISI

rarer types of disseminated encephalomyelitis – the chronic, recurrent (RDEM), and the multiphasic (MDEM) (Figure 49). The changes are of the same type as those seen in ADEM and may be the only means of differentiation from MS.

Other diseases which are frequently mistaken for MS on the basis of their MRI appearances include Lyme disease (Figure 50), HTLV-I-associated paraparesis (Figure 51), AIDS (Figure 52), cerebral arteritis such as lupus erythematosus, complicated migraine (Figure 53), trauma

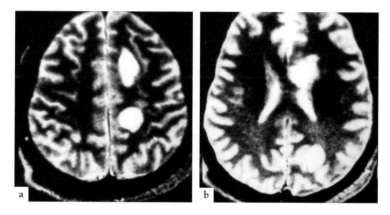

Figure 49 (a–f) Axial MRIs of a 29-year-old man with multiphasic disseminated encephalomyelitis (MDEM). The patient had a rapidly progressing right hemiparesis. The initial scan (a) revealed two large AISI in the left hemisphere, and a small one in the right hemisphere posteriorly. Biopsy of the left frontal AISI revealed inflammation and demyelination. AISI of this size are typical of ADEM. The patient recovered without treatment within 4 months. A follow-up scan taken 6 months later (b) showed shrinkage of the AISI and, 1 year later (c), two small AISI were all that remained. Three years later, following a flu-like illness, the patient complained of a moderately severe left hemiparesis. MRI at that time (d) showed a large new AISI in the right frontal area. A follow-up study 2 weeks later (e) showed what appeared to be reactivation of the two left hemisphere AISI despite the absence of right-sided symptoms. The patient recovered after treatment with methylprednisolone. A final scan 3 months later (f) showed considerable regression of all AISI. This case is a good example of the value of MRI in ruling out multiple sclerosis in a patient whose history is compatible with such a diagnosis. Courtesy of Dr Saeed Bohlega, King Faisal Specialists Hospital, Riyadh, Saudi Arabia; modified from Khan *et al.*, 1995 (*continued on page 76*)

(Figures 54, 55), cerebrovascular disease (Figure 56), neurosarcoidosis (Figure 57), and chronic fatigue syndrome (CFS). This last syndrome, occurring mostly in young women, shares with MS the same characteristic fatigue as well as some of the more typical symptoms and signs. In contrast, the following symptoms are useful in establishing the diagnosis of CFS rather than MS: migratory myalgia, arthralgia and painful paresthesias, sleep disturbance, anhedonia, and unusual and paradoxical reactions to medications (Figure 58).

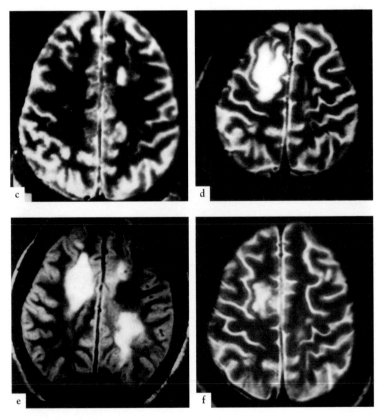

Figure 49 *Continued*

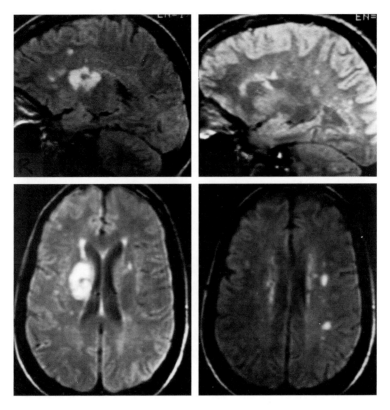

Figure 50 Coronal (upper) and axial (lower) proton density MRIs of a patient with Lyme disease show large periventricular areas of increased signal intensity similar to those seen in ADEM. Courtesy of Dr Patricia Hibberd, Massachusetts General Hospital, Boston, MA

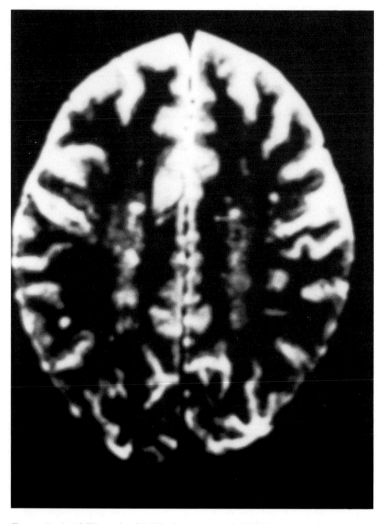

Figure 51 Axial T2-weighted MRI of a patient with HTLV-1-associated paraparesis. Courtesy of Dr Gustavo Roman, San Antonio, TX

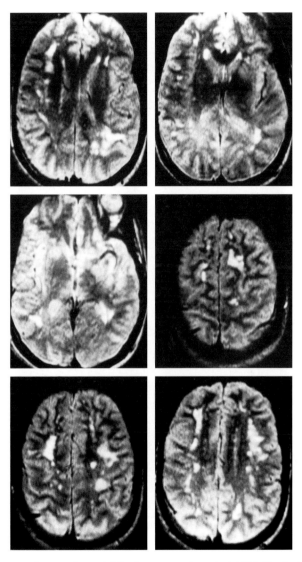

Figure 52 Axial proton-density MRIs of a patient with cerebral AIDS. Nearly all of the lesions lie at the periphery rather than in the periventricular area; this pattern is similar to that seen in ADEM

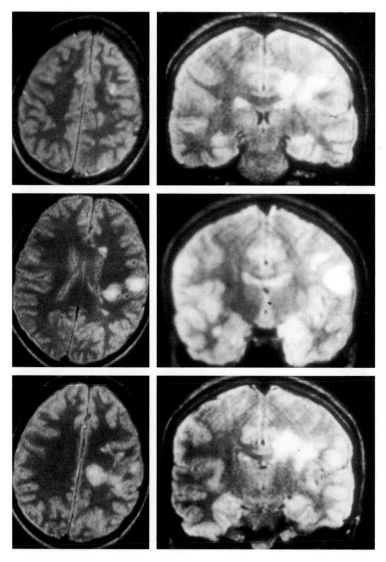

Figure 53 Axial (left) and coronal (right) proton-density MRIs of a patient who had complicated migraine. The pattern is similar to that seen in ADEM. Large cortical areas of increased signal intensity can be seen

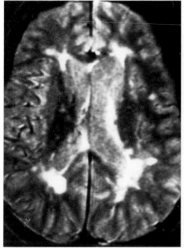

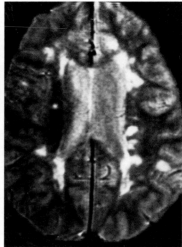

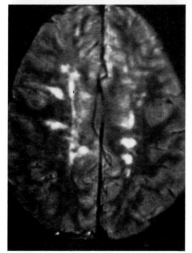

Figure 54 Axial proton-density MRI of a 42-year-old man who had suffered head trauma, specifically, a concussion. The patient complained of triple vision in the right eye and anxiety attacks. He had bilateral Babinski's signs, but had no other neurological symptoms or signs. He was diagnosed as having multiple sclerosis on the basis of the MRI. Note the markedly enlarged left ventricle. Further history disclosed that he had been comatose for a month after a car accident several years earlier

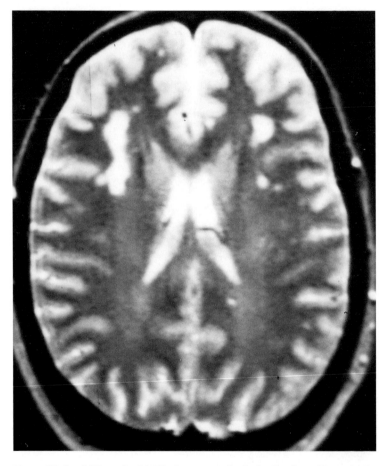

Figure 55 Axial T2-weighted MRI of a patient who had suffered a mild concussion without loss of consciousness. His only complaint was headache. Multiple areas of increased signal intensity are present in the cerebral white matter

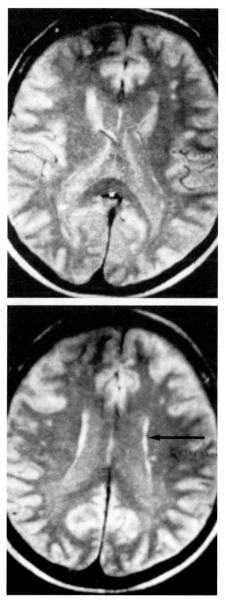

Figure 56 Axial proton-density MRIs of a patient with hypertensive cerebrovascular disease (Binswanger's) show scattered punctate and linear periventricular areas of increased signal intensity (arrow)

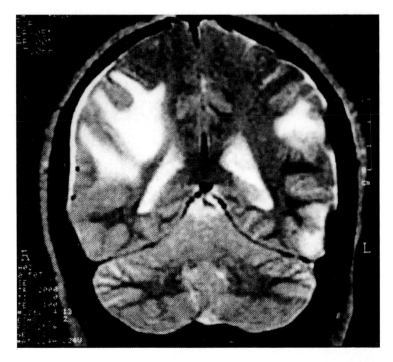

Figure 57 Coronal T2-weighted MRI of a patient with neurosarcoidosis. The lobar areas of increased signal intensity are similar to those seen in ADEM (see also Figure 47). Increased signal intensity of the meninges is highly characteristic

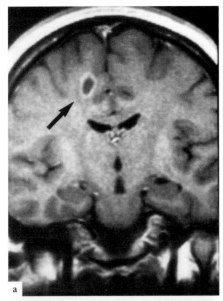

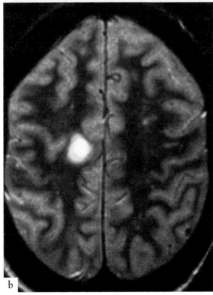

Figure 58 a and b T1-weighted MRI using gadolinium–EDTA injection (a) and proton-density MRI (b) of a patient with chronic fatigue syndrome (CFS). An enhancing lesion in the right parasagittal frontal cortex (a, arrow) corresponded to the patient's left-sided Babinski's sign. Despite the presence of neurological abnormalities, the patient fulfilled the diagnostic criteria for CFS

Single-photon emission computed tomography

Single-photon emission computed tomography (SPECT) uses radioactive tracers with computerized reconstruction of the isotopic emission recorded by a rotating gamma camera to measure cerebral perfusion. The applicability of SPECT to MS is limited to specialized research (Figure 59).

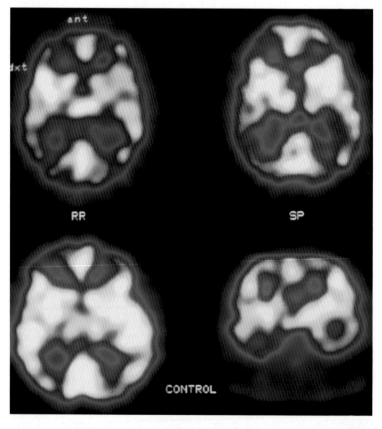

Figure 59 SPECT of the brain, using technetium-99 hexamethylpropyleneamine oxime, of two multiple sclerosis patients (upper) compared with a control (lower). Both patients clearly show a reduction in perfusion. Courtesy of Dr Jan Lycke, Sahlgrenska University Hospital, Göteborg, Sweden. For technical details, see Lycke *et al.*, 1993

Positron emission tomography

Using radiolabeled deoxyglucose, positron emission tomography (PET) has been reported to show as much as a 20–30% reduction in oxygen or glucose consumption in various parts of the brain in MS patients. PET is a research tool and requires close proximity to a cyclotron (Figures 60, 61).

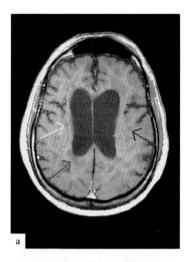

a

Figure 60 Axial post-gadolinium T1-weighted (a, b) and T2-weighted (c) MRIs, overlaid by cobalt–PET displays. Areas of non-enhancing hypodensity seen in (a) (arrow). Cobalt–PET-enhanced lesions may coincide (yellow and red arrows), but long-standing confluent lesions are neither enhanced nor show cobalt uptake (blue arrows). There is an enhanced lesion in (b) (magenta arrow) which does not show cobalt uptake. In general, there is good, but not complete, correlation between disease activity (gadolinium-enhanced) and cobalt–PET-enhanced lesions. Unpublished results, courtesy of H. Jansen, D. de Coo, J. De Reuck, J. Korf and J. Minderhoud, Groningen, The Netherlands, and Ghent, Belgium; courtesy of Dr Jakob Korf, University Hospital, Groningen, The Netherlands. For technical details, see Jansen *et al.*, 1995

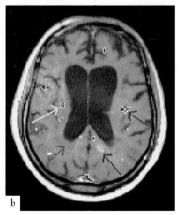

b

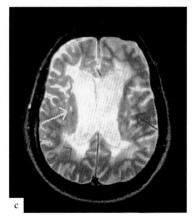

c

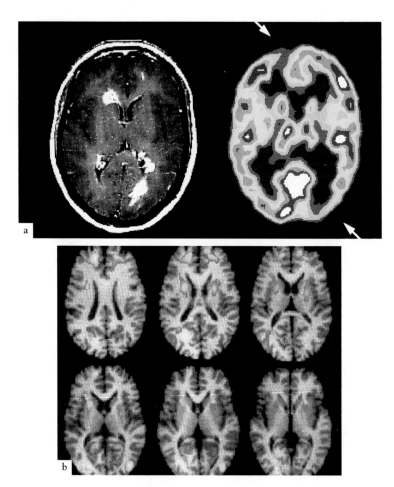

Figure 61 Axial contrast-enhanced MRI (a, left) compared with an ^{18}F-labeled deoxyglucose (FDG)–PET scan (a, right) of the brain. The color scale represents glucose consumption from 0 (black) to 45 (white) mol/100 ml/min. Areas of abnormal cortical glucose consumption (arrows) may be considered a consequence of the subcortical demyelinating lesions seen on the MRI. The significantly ($p = 0.005$) lower differences of glucose metabolism in multiple sclerosis patients with ($n = 19$) *vs* without ($n = 16$) fatigue are superimposed on axial MRIs of a healthy subject (b). Differences are most prominent in the frontal cortex, striatum and adjacent white matter. Courtesy of Drs U. Roelcke and K. Leenders, Paul Scherrer Institute, Villigen, Switzerland; from Roelcke *et al.*, 1997; reproduced with permission of Lippincott-Raven (b)

Treatment

Details of acute and long-term treatment of MS are beyond the scope of this volume. Five drugs have won government approval (in the United States). Three of them are forms of β-interferon (Avonex®, Betaseron®, Rebif®), one is a mixture of amino acids (Copaxone®), and one is an immunosuppressant (Novantrone®). Other drugs such as aza-thioprine are in wide use, especially in Europe. All of them reduce the frequency of relapses and of new T2-weighted and enhancing lesions on MRI in relapsing and remitting and secondary progressive MS. No clear-cut evidence has emerged to suggest that any of them significantly delays the progression of the disease.

Conclusion

Despite major gaps in our knowledge of the pathogenesis, epidemiology and genetics of multiple sclerosis, much progress has been made, not only in those areas of research, but also in refining confirmatory laboratory diagnostic procedures and improving methods of symptomatic treatment. Therapeutic trials for long-term treatment have shown encouraging results, but as yet unproved results over the long term. What remains unchallenged is the primary role played by the astute and experienced clinician in the diagnosis and treatment of the disease.

Bibliography

Books

Abramsky O, Ovadia H. *Frontiers in Multiple Sclerosis: Clinical Research and Therapy.* London: Martin Dunitz, 1997

Compston A, Ebers G, Lassmann H, Matthews B, Wekerle H, eds. *McAlpine's Multiple Sclerosis.* London: Churchill Livingstone, 1998

Paty D, Ebers G. *Multiple Sclerosis.* Philadelphia: F.A. Davis, 1998

Siva A, Kesselring J, Thompson A, eds. *Frontiers in Multiple Sclerosis, Volume 2.* London: Martin Dunitz, 1999

Journals

Adams C, Poston R, Buk S, et al. Inflammatory vasculitis in multiple sclerosis. *J Neurol Sci* 1985;69:269–83

Allen I, McQuaid S, Mirakhur M, et al. Pathological abnormalities in the normal appearing white matter in multiple sclerosis. *J Neurol Sci* 2001;22:141–4

American Academy of Ophthalmology. Intermediate uveitis. In *Basic and Clinical Science Course, Section 9: Intraocular Inflammation and Uveitis.* San Francisco: American Academy of Ophthalmology, 1997–1998:102

Barnes D, Munro P, Youl B, et al. The long-standing MS lesion. *Brain* 1991;114:1271–80

Benedikz J, Stefánsson M, Gudmundsson J, et al. The natural history of untreated multiple sclerosis in Iceland. *Clin Neurol Neurosurg* 2002;104:208–10

Brain R, Wilkinson M. The association of cervical spondylosis and disseminated sclerosis. *Brain* 1957;80:456–78

Brinar V. The differential diagnosis of multiple sclerosis. *Clin Neurol Neurosurg* 2002;104:211–20

Brody J, Sever J, Henson T. Virus antibody titers in multiple sclerosis patients, siblings and controls. *J Am Med Assoc* 1971;216:1441–6

Broman T. Supravital analysis of disorders in the cerebral vascular permeability. II. Two cases of multiple sclerosis. *Acta Psychiat Neurol Scand* 1947;46(Suppl):58–71

Cannella B, Raine C. The adhesion molecule and cytokine profile of multiple sclerosis lesions. *Ann Neurol* 1995;37:424–35

Chen C-J, Ro L-S, Chang C-N, *et al*. Serial MRI studies in pathologically verified Balo's concentric sclerosis. *J Comput Assist Tomogr* 1996;20:732–5

Compston A, Coles A. Multiple sclerosis. *Lancet* 2002;359:1221–31

Dawson J. The histology of disseminated sclerosis. *Trans R Soc Edinburgh* 1916;50:517–740

Dean G, Kurtzke J. On the risk of acquiring multiple sclerosis according to age at immigration to South Africa. *Br Med J* 1971;3:725–9

Ebers G, Kukay K, Bulman D, *et al*. A full genome search in multiple sclerosis. *Nat Genet* 1996;13:472–6

Fazekas F, Offenbacher H, Fuchs S, *et al*. Criteria for an increased specificity of MRI interpretation in elderly subjects with suspected multiple sclerosis. *Neurology* 1988;38:1822–5

Filippi M. Non-conventional MR techniques to monitor the evolution of multiple sclerosis. *Neurol Sci* 2001;22:195–200

Firth D. *The Case of Augustus d'Esté*. Cambridge: Cambridge University Press, 1948

Gay F, Drye T, Dick G, *et al*. The application of multifactorial cluster analysis in the staging of plaques in early multiple sclerosis. Identification and characterization of the primary demyelinating lesion. *Brain* 1997;120:1461–83

Gay F, Esiri M. Blood–brain barrier damage in acute multiple sclerosis plaques. *Brain* 1991;114:557–72

Gharagozloo A, Poe L, Collins G. Antemortem diagnosis of Baló's concentric sclerosis: correlative MR imaging and pathologic findings. *Radiology* 1994;191:817–9

Gonsette R, André-Balisaux G, Delmotte R. La perméabilité des vaisseaux cérébraux. IV. Démyélinisation expérimentale provoquée par des substances agissant sur la barrière hématoencéphalique. *Acta Neurol Belg* 1966;66:247–62

Hickey W. Migration of hematogenous cells through the blood–brain barrier and the initiation of CNS inflammation. *Brain Pathol* 1991;1:97–105

Jahnke U, Fischer F, Alvord E. Sequence homology between certain viral proteins and proteins related to encephalomyelitis and neuritis. *Science* 1985;229:282–4

Jansen H, Willemsen A, Sinnige L, *et al.* Cobalt-55 positron emission tomography in relapsing-progressive multiple sclerosis. *J Neurol Sci* 1995;132:139–45

Johnson M, Lavin P, Whetsell W Jr. Fulminant monophasic multiple sclerosis, Marburg's type. *J Neurol Neurosurg Psychiatry* 1990:53:918–21

Keltner J, Johnson C, Spurr J, *et al.* Baseline visual field profile of optic neuritis. *Arch Ophthalmol* 1993:111:231–4

Kesselring J, Miller D, Robb S, *et al.* Acute disseminated encephalomyelitis: MRI findings and distinction from multiple sclerosis. *Brain* 1990;113:291–302

Khan S, Yaqub B, Poser C, *et al.* Multiphasic encephalomyelitis presenting as alternating hemiplegia. *J Neurol Neurosurg Psychiatry* 1995;58:467–70

Kinnunen E, Valle M, Piiranen L, *et al.* Viral antibodies in MS: a nationwide co-twin study. *Arch Neurol* 1990:47:743–6

Kirk J. The fine structure of the CNS in multiple sclerosis. II. Vesicular demyelination in an acute case. *Neuropathol Appl Neurobiol* 1979;5:289–94

Kurtzke J, Gudmundsson K, Bergmann S. Multiple sclerosis in Iceland. I. Evidence of a postwar epidemic. *Neurology* 1982;32:143–50

Kurtzke J, Hyllested J. Multiple sclerosis in the Faroe Islands. I. Clinical and epidemiological features. *Ann Neurol* 1979;5:6–21

Lycke J, Wikkelsö C, Bergh A-C, *et al*. Regional cerebral blood flow in multiple sclerosis measured by single-photon emission tomography with technetium-99m hexamethyl propyleneamine oxime. *Eur Neurol* 1993;33:163–7

McDonald W, Compston A, Edan G, *et al*. Recommended diagnostic criteria for multiple sclerosis. *Ann Neurol* 2001;50:121–7

Miller A, Galboiz Y. Multiple sclerosis: from basic immunopathology to immune intervention. *Clin Neurol Neurosurg* 2002;104:172–4

Namerow N, Thompson L. Plaques, symptoms and the remitting course of multiple sclerosis. *Neurology* 1969;19:765–74

O'Connor P and the Canadian MS Working Group. Key issues in the diagnosis and treatment of multiple sclerosis. *Neurology* 2002;59(Suppl 3):S1–33

Olsson T, Sun J, Solders G, *et al*. Autoreactive T and B cell responses to myelin antigens after diagnostic sural nerve biopsy. *J Neurol Sci* 1993;117:130–9

Oppenheimer D. The cervical cord in multiple sclerosis. *Neuropathol Appl Neurobiol* 1978;4:151–62

Orrell R, Shakir R, Lane R, *et al*. Distinguishing acute disseminated encephalomyelitis from multiple sclerosis. *Br Med J* 1996;313:802–4

Paty D, Poser C. Clinical symptoms and signs of multiple sclerosis. In Poser C, Paty D, Scheinberg L, *et al*., eds. *The Diagnosis of Multiple Sclerosis*. New York: Thieme-Stratton, 1984:27–43

Poser C. Exacerbations, activity and progression in multiple sclerosis. *Arch Neurol* 1980;37:471–4

Poser C. The course of multiple sclerosis. *Arch Neurol* 1985;42:1035

Poser C. The pathogenesis of multiple sclerosis. A critical reappraisal. *Acta Neuropathol* 1986;71:1–10

Poser C. Magnetic resonance imaging in asymptomatic disseminated vasculomyelinopathy. *J Neurol Sci* 1989;94:69–7

Poser C. The epidemiology of multiple sclerosis. A general overview. *Ann Neurol* 1994;36(S 2):S180–93

Poser C. The role of trauma in the pathogenesis of multiple sclerosis. A review. *Clin Neurol Neurosurg* 1994;96:103–10

Poser C. Myalgic encephalomyelitis/chronic fatigue syndrome and multiple sclerosis: differential diagnosis. *EOS J lmmunol lmmunopharmacol* 1995;196:765–71

Poser C. Onset symptoms of multiple sclerosis. *J Neurol Neurosurg Psychiatry* 1995;58:253–4

Poser C. The pathogenesis of multiple sclerosis. *Clin Neurosci* 1994;2:258–65

Poser C. The pathogenesis of multiple sclerosis: a commentary. *Clin Neurol Neurosurg* 2000;102:191–4

Poser C, Brinar V. Problems with diagnostic criteria for multiple sclerosis. *Lancet* 2001;358:1746–7

Poser C, Brinar V. The symptomatic treatment of multiple sclerosis. *Clin Neurol Neurosurg* 2002;104:231–5

Poser C, Goutières F, Carpentier M-A, *et al.* Schilder's myelinoclastic diffuse sclerosis. *Pediatrics* 1986;77:107–12

Poser C, Hibberd P, Benedikz J, *et al.* An analysis of the "epidemic" of multiple sclerosis in the Faroe Islands. *Neuroepidemiology* 1988;7:168–80

Poser C, Paty D, Scheinberg L, *et al.* New diagnostic criteria for multiple sclerosis. *Ann Neurol* 1983;13:227–31

Poser C, Roman G, Vernant J-C. Multiple sclerosis or HTLV-I myelitis? *Neurology* 1990;40:1020–2

Pozzilli C, Bernardi S, Mansi U, et al. Quantitative assessment of blood–brain barrier permeability in multiple sclerosis using 68-Ga-EDTA and positron emission tomography. *J Neurol Neurosurg Psychiatry* 1988;51:1058–62

Pryse-Phillips W. New long-term treatments for multiple sclerosis. *Clin Neurol Neurosurg* 2002;104:265–71

Pugliatti M, Sotgiu S, Solinas G, et al. Multiple sclerosis prevalence among Sardinians: further evidence against the latitude gradient theory. *Neurol Sci* 2001;22:163–6

Raine C. The immunology of multiple sclerosis. *Ann Neurol* 1994;36:S61–72

Robertson N, Clayton D, Fraser M, et al. Clinical concordance in sibling pairs with multiple sclerosis. *Neurology* 1996;47:347–52

Roizin L, Helfand M, Moore J. Disseminated diffuse and transitional demyelination of the central nervous system. *J Nerv Ment Dis* 1946;104:1–50

Sadovnick A. The genetics of multiple sclerosis. *Clin Neurol Neurosurg* 2002;104:199–202

Sagar H, Warlow C, Sheldon P, et al. Multiple sclerosis with clinical and radiological features of cerebral tumour. *J Neurol Neurosurg Psychiatry* 1982;45:802–8

Sotgiu S, Pugliatti M, Solinas G. Immunogenetic heterogeneity of multiple sclerosis in Sardinia. *Neurol Sci* 2001;22:167–70

Wingerchuk D, Hogancamp W, O'Brien P, et al. The clinical course of neuromyelitis optica (Devic's syndrome). *Neurology* 1999;53:1107–14

Woyciechowska J, Dambrozia J, Chu A, et al. Correlation of oligoclonal IgG bands and viral antibodies in twins with multiple sclerosis. In Cazzullo C, Caputo D, Ghezze A, et al., eds. *Virology and Immunology in Multiple Sclerosis*. Berlin: Springer-Verlag, 1987:45–9

Index

abbau 25, 29

acoustic nerves 31

acute disseminated encephalomyelitis (ADEM) 25, 42, 68, 72, 74–75

adhesion molecules 21

age of acquisition 9–10

age of onset 8

AIDS 47, 75, 79

antibody response 13–21

antigenic challenge 13–21

areas of increased signal intensity (AISIs) 22, 59, 60–62, 68, 75

astrocytes, gemistocytic 25, 30

astrocytic gliosis 38

axonal damage 25, 35, 37–38, 68

azathioprine 89

β-interferon 89

B-lymphocytes 13, 14

Baló's disease 31, 32–33, 70

basal ganglia 31

Binswanger's disease 83

blood–brain barrier deficits 13, 14, 18–23

brain stem 25, 40, 56

  auditory responses 54, 69

burden of disease 59

burned-out MS 42

cerebellum 25, 40, 56, 58

cerebral arteritis 75

cerebral hemispheres 25–31

cerebrospinal fluid examination 47, 52

cerebrovascular disease 54, 76, 83

chronic fatigue syndrome (CFS) 76, 85

clinical aspects 40–44

clinical course 7–8, 22–23, 41–42

computed tomography (CT) 55–59

concentric alternating demyelination 31, 32–33

concordance, in monozygotic twins 11, 13

concussion 81–82

course of disease 7–8, 22–23, 41–42

cranial nerves 31

cystoid macular edema 50

cytokines 21

demyelination 22–23, 27, 31, 35–38, 68

  concentric alternating 31, 32–33

  see also myelinoclasia

dentate nuclei 26, 31

Devic's disease 31

diagnosis 44–88

  confirmatory laboratory procedures 45–55

    evoked potential studies 53–55

    lumbar puncture 47

    see also neuroimaging

  diagnostic criteria 44–45

    new diagnostic criteria of McDonald 45, 46, 59

diffuse sclerosis 31, 34

disease course 7–8, 22–23, 41–42

disk herniation 60, 64

disseminated encephalomyelitis *see* encephalomyelitis

edema 21, 22, 31
  cystoid macular edema 50
encephalomyelitis
  disseminated 47, 75
    acute (ADEM) 25, 42, 68, 72, 74–75
    multiphasic (MDEM) 47, 75
    recurrent (RDEM) 47, 71, 75
  postvaccination 73
environmental influence 11
epidemics 9–10
epidemiology 9–11
etiology 12
evoked potential studies 53, 54

facial nerve 31
facial palsy 68
familial occurrence 11
fibrinogen leakage 18–19

gadolinium-enhanced MRI 60–65
gemistocytic astrocytes 25, 30
genetics 10–11, 13
geographical variation 9–10
glaucoma 54
glial scars 23, 25
gliosis 27, 68
  astrocytic 38

head trauma 81–82
herniated disks 60, 64
HTLV-I-associated paraparesis 47, 75, 78
human leukocyte antigen (HLA) system 10–11
hypothalamus 31

immune complexes 21
inflammation 22, 25, 68
internuclear ophthalmoplegia 31, 54

laboratory tests *see* diagnosis
lumbar puncture 47
lupus erythematosus 75
Lyme disease 47, 75, 77
lymphocytic infiltration 13, 17, 21

McDonald diagnostic criteria 45, 46, 59
macrophages 25, 29, 31, 35–36, 38
magnetic resonance imaging (MRI) 59–68
  gadolinium enhancement 60–65
major histocompatibility complex (MHC) 10–11
Marburg disease 42
median longitudinal fasciculus 31
migraine, complicated 75, 80
molecular mimicry 21
monozygotic twins, concordance 11, 13
MS trait (MST) 13–21
multiphasic disseminated encephalomyelitis (MDEM) 47, 75
myelin abbau 25, 29
myelin sheath 39
  see also demyelination; myelinoclasia; remyelination
myelinoclasia 22, 29, 42–43
  see also demyelination

neuroimaging 55–88
  computed tomography (CT) 55–59
  imaging differential diagnoses 68–85
  magnetic resonance imaging (MRI) 59–68

positron emission tomography (PET) 87–88
  single-photon emission computed tomography (SPECT) 86
neuromyelitis optica 31
neurosarcoidosis 76, 84
neurosyphilis 47
nodes of Ranvier 39

oligoclonal bands 13, 14, 52
oligodendrocytes 22, 37
onset
  age at 8
  symptoms 40
optic atrophy 49, 51, 54, 56
optic chiasm 31, 40, 53
optic fundus 45
optic nerve 31, 40, 45, 49, 53
optic neuritis 15, 51, 67

papillitis 48
parenchymatous lesions 26
pathogenesis 13–24
pathology 25–38
periphlebitis 50
periventricular lesions 26–27, 38
physiology 39
plaques 14, 19–20, 25, 27–28, 30, 39
  features of 42
  formation 40
  neuroimaging 58, 59–60
  Schilder's disease 34
  shadow plaques 27
  spinal cord 58, 59–60, 66
pons 28

positron emission tomography (PET) 87–88
postvaccination encephalomyelitis 73
prevalence 9
  geographical variation 9–10
primary progressive MS (PPMS) 41, 45
pseudo-Baló's disease 71
pseudo-exacerbations 39

Raine, Cedric 23
reactive gliosis 27
recurrent disseminated encephalomyelitis (RDEM) 47, 71, 75
relapsing and remitting MS (RRMS) 41
remyelination 7, 21–23, 27, 31, 38

safety factor 42, 43
saltatory conduction 39
sarcoidosis 47
Schilder's disease 31, 34
scotoma 51
secondary progressive MS (SPMS) 41
shadow plaques 27
signs 39, 40, 41
single-photon emission computed tomography (SPECT) 86
somatosensory evoked responses 55
spinal cord 25, 28, 31, 40
  compression 59–60, 64–65
  plaques 58, 59–60, 66
  whiplash injury 66
spondylosis 40, 59, 65
symptoms 39, 40, 41

T-lymphocytes 21
thalamus 31